A VEGAN PLANET

Your guide to a life transforming journey

JEFF LETENDRE

ISBN: 978-107748-296-8

"The only thing necessary for evil to triumph is for good men to do nothing."

Edmund Burke

CONTENTS

ACKNOWLEDGEMENTS

I would like to thank my girlfriend, family, friends, and co-workers who have encouraged me to write this book and supported me through so many past adventures. You know who you are. Without you by my side, many of my crazy projects would not have been possible. Being busy with my daily activities, I may not have thanked you enough or as often as I wished: thanks, from the bottom of my heart.

I would also like to acknowledge the millions of animal lovers who have made veganism the movement it is today. I would like to express my respect and gratitude to those who have pioneered the animal rights movement. I would like to thank all organizations, groups, and individuals who are not only voicing their concerns but defending the powerless victims in the hands of humanity's darker side.

I would like to thank the great minds behind vegan companies developing cruelty-free products of the present and future. I would like to thank celebrities, politicians, athletes, artists, and scientists who are using their influence to promote animal rights.

I would like to thank my two adorable Jack Russells Suki,

and Solo who are teaching me daily just how insightful, emotional, and loving animals are.

Finally, I would like to acknowledge the billions of animals who are enslaved or suffering in cages around the world. I acknowledge your screams for justice and compassion. I acknowledge your longing for freedom and your right to live in peace. I acknowledge you, like the thousands of activists trying to end your exploitation. We see you. We hear you. A more compassionate world is coming soon.

FOREWORD

By **Xavier Desharnais**,
Professional Marathon Swimmer

"You must eat meat."
"Plant protein is not like animal protein."
"Eat a good steak before the race, just to be sure."

I heard it all during my first few years as a high-level vegan athlete. I became vegan in 2012 because I wanted to enhance my performance and get ahead of my opponents. At an international level, every good athlete trains similarly. I was looking for a way to optimize my training, to do something no other swimmers were doing. Through my search, I read a lot of science and concluded that a plant-based diet could be a means of bringing me to the next level.

In my beginnings, people believed my new lifestyle would be short-lived. They said I would give up within three months, one year, three years maximum. Nobody imagined my plant-based diet could last, especially in the high-level sports world, where steak and chicken are kings.

After a few good results in the first year; 1st World Cup podium and personal best times, I had a rougher second year. Even though I managed to climb on the second step of a World Cup podium again, I was told it was most likely because I used to eat meat, and if I had continued that way, I could have taken the first place.

For an athlete who is always aiming for perfection, having doubts can be brutal. Swimming is a lonely sport. You train and compete on your own and spend a lot of time in your head. Swimming in silence looking at a big black line at the bottom of a pool for 30 hours a week is difficult enough, you don't need external pressure about your diet.

Regardless, I stayed the course, and it was finally in 2014 that I last heard someone suggest I eat a little bit of meat before the race. It was the last time because it was the year I became the first Canadian swimmer in 20 years to win the famous Traversée Internationale du Lac St-Jean, a 32km swim across Lac St-Jean, in Quebec Canada. This race is one of the most grueling and challenging endurance events in the world.

Now being the fastest in the world to swim 32km across a cold-water lake, with waves reaching up to six feet, who would dare tell me I needed animal protein? It was also at this exact moment that my doubts disappeared forever, and that I knew I had found my secret weapon: a 100% plant-based power supply!

Today, at seven years being vegan, I have seen the many benefits it provides. Not only did it help my sports performance, but I have found myself significantly reducing my impact on the environment, on top of saving thousands of animal lives.

Since 2012, the year I became vegan, I saved over 10,000,000 liters of freshwater, 45,000 kg of grain, 7,000 square meters of forest, 23,000 kg of CO2 and 2,500 animal lives.[1]

Though my athletic career is over, I would still not go back to eating meat and by-products in everyday life. If there is one thing I regret, it's not starting a vegan diet earlier!

I sincerely hope Jeff's book will give you a different view on veganism and debunk some of the myths related to animal consumption. Don't we say we are what we eat?

---

[1] https://thevegancalculator.com

INTRODUCTION

I used to be a meat-eater. I used to hunt, fish, and trap. My mom still has earmuffs made from beaver fur I caught myself. I had pets and loved spending time in the wild. I considered myself an animal and nature lover. I ate meat multiple times a day. Animal consumption was part of my everyday life. I never questioned my relationship with animals.

That all changed the day I read the book "Awaken the Giant Within" by Tony Robbins back in 1998, when I was 19 years old. There was a chapter on veganism, the environment, and industrial animal farming. Upon finishing the book, I went to my fridge and gave away all the meat, fish, and dairy I had. Learning about veganism was an eye-opener for me. While I saw myself as an animal lover, I realized that my actions did not reflect this belief.

Years went by and I did my best to convince people around me to consider veganism, but those conversations usually brought up a few minutes of empathy without any follow-up. Though frustrating and sad, I accepted there wasn't much more I could do.

In recent years, my social media feed constantly displayed pictures and videos of animals suffering in factory farms, ocean pollution, massive deforestation, dying wildlife, industrial fishing, and climate change just to name a few. A harsh daily reminder of what humans are capable of and what a senseless situation we have put our ecosystem in.

What kept me up at night, what disturbed me the most, was not necessarily the result of our actions, but knowing the solution to end this nightmare was so obvious, and so easy to do. Even though I consider myself an optimist, on some days, it became an exasperating burden to live with. How can we be so cruel, and, quite frankly, dumb? How can the most intelligent species on Earth cause its own downfall while the solutions are right there, ready to be implemented?

For such blatant ignorance, I could not stand idle anymore. I had to do more than talking or posting to help our planet and the animals. While I never intended to be a writer, writing this book was something I felt I could do to have more of an impact. Afterall, having been a vegan for over twenty years, I have gathered a lot of information on the subject.

Even though it's not easy to remain positive in the face of so much complacency, I know most of us care about the destruction of the environment and animal cruelty. One explanation behind our society's behavior are the years and billions of dollars invested by the meat industry's marketing campaigns. They have taught us to turn a blind eye and accept the unacceptable.

As part of my recent training, I was doing a long-distance bike ride between Montreal and my hometown city, Drummondville. Farmland represents 80% of the 100km separating the 2 cities. One would think it would have been a beautiful relaxing sight biking through lush organic green fields, animal pasture, and archetypical farms, but the reality was shockingly different.

The first thing to hit you is the stench of animal feces from the buildings where thousands of sentient beings are held captive. Fields of manure filled the air for kilometers among the streams and rivers polluted with fertilizing chemicals and pesticides. I can still smell it now as I write this.

It has been a while since I had ventured into the countryside and I was amazed by the industrialization and normalization of such a system. Most animal factory farms have a logo of smiling pigs, cows, or chickens at the entrance. What a deceitful statement when you look at the windowless sheds in the background where animal slaves are forced bred and kept in terrible conditions.

On one of the pig farms I passed, the corpse of a big hog was left outside by the shed, bloated under the sun, like a piece of trash. As the body didn't show any sign of injuries, one can only imagine the conditions and sickness this animal must have endured before dying.

The sight of these factories reminded me of concentration camps. Let's not be afraid of using the right terms here, these installations are nothing short of gulags of despair for the animal victims trapped inside. Comparing concentration camps with factory farms only seems like an exaggeration where cruelty is normalized. If you disagree, I invite you to visit a factory farm and decide for yourself. You'll discover a vision of hell.

Desensitized from the way our food is produced, we no longer see the animal behind our hot-dog sausages. And even when we recognize the cruelty, many doubt what difference one human could have. Why bother trying veganism when almost everyone else is eating meat and dairy?

Social psychology refers to this phenomenon as "social proof." The proof of what is right and acceptable is provided by the behavior and actions of numerous people. The higher the number of people who find a habit or tradition to be acceptable, the more correct and valid the habit will be no matter how ruthless, vile, or destructive.

Very few are willing to go against the majority and question the foundations of what millions are endorsing. What is key to remember is that what is popular isn't always right, and what is right isn't always popular.

Humanity has seen a never-ending stream of cultural, political, and religious revolutions. Slavery, segregation, and colonialism are all examples of oppressive systems that are no longer acceptable but used to be the norm in many societies.

German philosopher **Arthur Schopenhauer** once said:

"All truth passes through three stages. First it is ridiculed, second, it is violently opposed. Third, it is accepted as being self-evident."

Throughout history, leaders challenging the norm were often not taken seriously or seen as trying to push their beliefs onto others. Think of first abolition movement activist William Lloyd Garrison, Civil rights movement activist Martin Luther King, peaceful independence activist Mohandas Gandhi, the early feminists or unionists from the 19th century. All of them faced tremendous resistance in the early stages of their historical movements. Today we can draw a parallel between past and contemporary activists. Most of the population still rejects veganism and its chances of becoming the norm.

It is difficult to understand why seemingly obvious, progressive evolutions were met with such hostility and opposition. Though it may seem like humanity is progressing, our current response to animal cruelty is a reminder that while the victims have changed, our modern society perpetuates the same level of brutality as centuries ago.

Even if a plant-based world seems out of reach, let's remind ourselves of **Victor Hugo**'s words:

"Nothing is more powerful and unstoppable than a great idea which time has come."

The fight ahead looks as formidable as any other before, but we must rise to the challenge. Veganism is key to not only our own survival and evolution, but to the planet's ecosystem. The status quo is no longer an option.

My main objective with this book is to help raise awareness to the cause and to the desperate call of our animal friends stuck in cages across the globe. I hope to help reconnect as many as possible with feelings of compassion and common sense that years of corporate propaganda has buried within us.

As children, each of us were true animal lovers and activists but along the way, we have learned to accept their killing for fashion or flavors. We have learned to accept the imprisonment of animals for entertainment and experiments. We have learned to treat them as slaves, as disposable objects. Truth is, we have been fooled; we have been lied to.

It is time to question ourselves, the systems we live and participate in, and rebuild our relationship with the ecosystem we are part of. We undoubtedly can make veganism the most peaceful, impactful revolution of our history.

A vegan planet is anything but a utopia, it is the one chance we have at resolving global warming and reshaping our future into something beautiful and exciting for all.

1. THE MEANING OF VEGANISM

A plant-based diet, which is often referred to as a vegan diet, means a diet exempt of any animal products: meat, fish, seafood, eggs, dairy, and honey. At first, it might be difficult to imagine what is left on the table to eat, but later in the book, we'll see how easy it is nowadays to have a delicious, balanced and varied plant-based diet.

When we are talking about veganism, it is much broader than a simple diet. It is a way of life where one puts compassion and common sense before personal gain, pleasure, or habits. Food is one important element, but veganism applies to the use of any animal by-products or animal exploitation such as; leather, wool, fur, dawn, horse carriages, animal testing in labs, using animals in circus, etc.

A taste of a few seconds in someone's mouth, a custom or a religious ceremony is less important than an animal's suffering and life. It is based on this logic that vegans refrain from causing needless pain and torment to sentient beings who want to live just as much as we do.

There is no fundamental difference between humans and animals in their ability to feel pleasure and pain, happiness, and misery. Anyone with pets at home will agree animals have their own personalities. They can feel lonely, they can feel stress, happiness, and excitement just to name a few emotions they have in common with us. Animals imprisoned in industrial complexes are no different than our cats or dogs we cherish and protect. Why should we treat them any different? Why eat them when non-essential to our health and survival?

As for animal exploitation, a vegan would not buy a ticket for Sea World. The dolphins and orcas are taken away from their families and freedom to entertain humans. It is psychological torture to keep these animals captive in tiny concrete pools when they are meant to freely roam the ocean. The kisses and water splashes may look fun to the crowd, but these intelligent mammals are forced to learn special tricks in order to eat or cope with extreme boredom. They may seem to enjoy giving a show, but studies have demonstrated they all suffer from some form of depression or anxiety.

The same principles apply to leather and fur. Why force breed or trap gentle creatures to wear their skin for fashion or trend? Whenever questioning if a practice is right or not, just ask yourself if you would like to have it done to you. If the answer is no, most likely, the animal feels just the same.

Our overwhelming power and condescending attitude toward anything non-human, does not give us the right to abuse animals with such carelessness.

Many will say humans are apex predators, just like lions. They will say nature is cruel, and the strong eats the weak. Why wouldn't humans follow nature's law and do what carnivorous predators do in the wild?

The truth is, we have absolutely nothing in common with

carnivores. Not the strength, not the speed, not the teeth, not the claws, and not the digestive system to digest animal corpses. I don't recall any humans ever being attracted to the smell of a decaying zebra that lions have been feeding on for days.

Human teeth have way more similarity to a horse's dentition than any meat-eaters. Carnivores do not chew their food; they do not have molar teeth. They cut their food in pieces and swallow it in chunks. Our mini canines, which for some is a proof of our omnivore status, would be of no help in killing or cutting open a dead furry body.

Could you imagine tearing a rabbit's skin with your mouth? We can hardly chew on a fresh, clean, thoroughly cooked steak, and some would believe we should compare ourselves with top predators like lions. In fact, eating any parts of a lion or bear's catch without quickly cooking it would make us very sick, or worse, send us to our death.

Nature gives equal chances to both the zebra and the lions to survive. There is a perfect balance between the zebra's capacity to escape, and the lion's ability to catch its prey. There is no such balance when a cow is chained to the slaughterhouse's conveyor belt. Nature's law does not imply building massive farming industrial complexes, hunting with guns or fishing the ocean with trawlers.

Today we are mostly cut off from the natural world, our modern way of life is very different from our ancestors. We cannot excuse ourselves with such arguments and perpetuate our actions, thinking it is natural, when we are, in fact, destroying nature.

If I were living in the wild centuries ago, I would obviously use every resource at my disposition to survive, including hunting. Cooking and eating fresh meat became a huge factor in our survival by expanding our limited food supply during that time.

Nowadays, with 7 billion humans walking the Earth, our everyday life is not organized around physical survival anymore. Hunting has turned into a sport, a pastime purely based on leisure.

Oceans are being emptied by fleets of trawler vessels catching entire schools of fish, destroying ecosystems, and stealing precious sources of food from sea animals.

Animal farming has gone completely mad. Sentient beings are called "livestock," which imply that they are no more than living merchandise and treated as such. They are raised in massive industrial complexes where living conditions are so horrific, we cannot even watch it on videos.

As for agriculture, the overuse of pesticide to yield as much as possible to feed 56 billion livestock has turned into an ecological disaster the world over.

As you can see, we are far, far away from our ancestor's way of life. It would be ludicrous to compare what was then a necessity to what is now nothing but destruction, cruelty, and human greed.

By any means, if we were able to look at ourselves and our behaviors, we would be called nothing short of a virus, we would be a "pest" to eliminate as quickly as possible. Everywhere you see humans, there is destruction, abuse, pollution, and selfishness toward the planet's ecosystem.

But it's not too late, we can learn, we can change, and we can act. This essentially what veganism is about. A study conducted by the University of Michigan called, "The environmental impact of the vegan beyond burger vs. a ¼ pound beef burger" revealed that the veggie burger will use 99% less water, 93% less land, 90% fewer greenhouse gas emissions and 46% less energy to produce.[2] Not to mention the veggie burger is packed with nutrients and tastes just the same.

We eat three times a day, that's over a thousand meals a year. Can you imagine the impact if the whole world was vegan? In a time where the threat of global warming is omnipresent, how on Earth could we not immediately make such a small change? We are only talking about a burger, but almost every dish has a vegan equivalent that tastes just like the meat version.

Soldiers go to war to defend their country's interests. Very often, these conflicts are complicated to understand or justify, yet, thousands of soldiers are ready to get to the battlefield. They are prepared to leave their families behind for months or years at a time, they are willing to take a bullet or lose their life for what politicians are telling them to do. It is their duty!

Don't we think we have a duty to save the ecosystem as we know it? Don't we have a duty to give our children a future? Don't we have a duty to love and protect our animal friends

---

[2] http://css.umich.edu/publication/beyond-meats-beyond-burger-life-cycle-assessment-detailed-comparison-between-plant-based (2018)

Aren't these missions important and noble enough? We don't have to go to war for this mission, we don't have to risk our lives or leave our loved ones behind. To fulfill our duty, to save the world, and our future, all we have to do is eat the veggie burger. Are we the most intelligent species on Earth?

2. WE ARE ALL ANIMALS

I was sitting at my cottage in the Laurentian mountains watching pair of wild mallard ducks eating grains I left on the riverbank. They were flying in together, at around the same time each day. They would always be next to each other, watching over each other while eating.

Looking at them, I was wondering about their daily routine. It was June, so the couple must have had chicks to look after. How were they communicating to raise their babies? When are they getting up, going to sleep? Who decides, the male or the female? How would they know where they were flying to?

It became very apparent to me that we are probably just unable to understand animal language. Think about it, when they are both flying in the air, how do they know their destination? If there were no grains left at my place, they would fly somewhere else or find other food from the river. But again, as they are a pair how do they know what they are doing? How do they communicate things like when to fly back to the nest? Which one decides the nest needs more branches or feathers to make it warmer for the chicks?

To us, "quack quack" are just noises, but it must contain complex information that we don't understand. After all, to them, humans make unintelligible noises from their mouths too.

These two ducks, they randomly met at some point and decided to mate and pair up. They searched and found a suitable location to build their nest. They found different sources of food. They protected themselves from the elements. The female laid eggs and covered them until they hatched. They fed and protected their chicks together until they were old enough to live on their own. Once the fall arrives, the ducks fly south thousands of kilometers showing amazing geolocation skills.

They have a full and complex life of their own. They communicate, have social and sexual interactions, they have friends, they build their own houses, they protect themselves from predators and the elements. They have a daily job finding food, they learn, memorize, travel, and raise their own offspring. Are they all so different from us?

The human mind is clearly extraordinary: animals don't compose symphonies, design aircraft, or devise experiments to probe one another's mental abilities. But how are we comparing ourselves to them? We got lucky, nature gave us the biggest brain of all, and it turned out to be the most successful tool to survive. If we base our studies to differentiate ourselves on cognitive tests alone, we will obviously win every time and easily outclass any other animals. But is it a fair test? How would a human rank against a bear if we were to design a similar analysis based on smell? Or an ultrasound test against an echolocating bat? Speed test against a cheetah? What if we tested a dog's loyalty compared to a human's? What about testing greed and compassion levels between animals and humans? Animals have much more to teach us than we think.

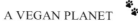

"We cannot judge a fish by its ability to climb a tree."

Albert Einstein

How would you react if in order to get your next job, at the interview, you were asked to be qualified in a completely different field than what you have studied for? Let's say you apply for a nursing position, but the employer asks you to be a fully qualified underwater welder. You would obviously not get the job, but would that make you an inferior candidate or a less intelligent one? No, you are good at nursing, and you rightfully know nothing about underwater welding.

It is a comparison we can make with animals. You can't ask a bird to design an aircraft, nor can you ask a human to fly. Our brain capacity, even though very helpful and empowering to us, should never be a reason to exploit, dominate, murder, or look down on other creatures that were simply given different talents to survive. Why not use our intelligence to help, support, and protect our animal friends with whom we are sharing the Earth?

3. VEGAN FOR THE ANIMALS

"The time will come when men such as I will look on the murder of animals as they now look on the murder of men."

Leonardo da Vinci

S ome people go vegan for health benefits in an effort to avoid, or cure diseases linked to meat consumption such as heart conditions, cancer, diabetes, harmful cholesterol, acne, and so on. On this subject, I suggest you watch the documentary, "What the Health". It is loaded with facts and impactful information that will have you think twice about your next non-vegan meal. I will get deeper into the health and biology side of veganism in a later chapter.

Health and fitness are noteworthy reasons to go vegan, but for myself and many early vegans, the driving forces of change are our love for the animals and the desire to end their suffering. I have no doubt most people would call themselves animal lovers, but they fail to make the connection between what they eat, wear, or get entertained by.

A good example is someone walking their dog wearing the popular Canada Goose jacket with a fur trim. If they take the time to go out for a walk, they must care and love their animal. Yet, they have paid for a product that force breeds and traps foxes and coyotes, cousins to dogs. The fur trim is nothing more than a fashion garment. Many alternatives exist to keep warm.

How would they feel if someone was trapping their dogs in their backyard to make a piece of fashion? The culprit would most likely make news headlines and be labeled as a psychopath. Yet, they buy and proudly wear the infamous Canada Goose jacket. This is the epitome of not making a connection between loving animals and exploiting them.

To hide the dark side of their products and fool customers, corporations are using deceiving marketing practices. It is easy to forget what lies behind the cute image of a smiling cow on a dairy product. Yet, we must see past the appearance and uncover the truth. Every single animal-based product involves some level of cruelty.

Free-range eggs, grass-fed cows, humanely killed, grain-fed chicken, sustainable fishing, organic meat are labels and practices designed for one thing; making you feel good and less guilty about your choices. There is no way to humanely rape, torture, or kill an animal just as there is no way to humanely rape, torture, or kill a human. Do not be fooled, the only reason behind ethical animal treatment labels is to create an illusion of welfare. It is designed to keep your money flowing into the pockets of corporations.

"I only eat chicken."

I often hear people say that they hardly eat meat, only chicken. Somehow it seems more ethical. It may be due to the recent popularity of the uncaged chicken or free-range labels designed to make people feel good about their purchase. Unfortunately, it is no more than a marketing scam. As it turns out, on top of more stress, the birds are exposed to higher levels of bacteria, parasites, and viruses that put them at greater risk of disease and infection compared to their caged counterparts.

Research conducted by Sweden's National Veterinary Institute, reveals the truth about free range chicken:

> Free-range chickens are often housed in shelters where the floor doubles as a giant litter box. As a result, hens have direct contact with bacteria and microorganisms that grow in the litter, which can greatly increase health risks. Considering the size of the populations in the different housing systems, a larger proportion of laying hens than expected was submitted for necropsy from litter-based systems and free-range production compared to hens in cages. The research results demonstrated a significantly higher occurrence of bacterial and parasitic diseases and cannibalism in laying hens kept in litter-based housing systems and free-range systems than in hens kept in cages. [3]

Either imprisoned in a tiny cage or packed on a giant litter box, chickens live a miserable life. There is no way around it, the only humane thing to do is not eat them or their eggs. Chickens are forced bred and live without fresh air, sunlight, rain, freedom, natural social interaction, possibility to spread their wings, or the ability to scratch the soil for insects or other food. Restrained in a space filled with ammonia gas,

---

[3] Causes of mortality in laying hens in different housing systems in 2001 to 2004 by Oddvar Fossum et al. Acta Veterinaria Scandinavica (2009)

feces, flies, and the deafening sound of thousands of birds, chickens are forced to produce eggs way past their natural capacity without ever seeing their chicks. They are genetically modified, sick, pumped with antibiotics and other medication to withstand such pollution and diseases. Have we gone mad?

"I only eat chicken" makes no more sense than "I only eat ham or beef". They suffer just as much as any other species, and anyone who has been in contact with chicken before knows they are smart and loving creatures. In terms of numbers, they are the most abused land animal, a staggering 40 billion broilers a year are bred in hellish conditions. With abundant and delicious alternatives, this massacre is entirely unnecessary.

"What's wrong with eggs?"

I could not talk about chicken without mentioning eggs. Many people argue eating eggs doesn't kill the hens and is, therefore, more acceptable. Let's think this through for a moment. Given the choice, would you rather be enslaved for a few months and be sent to a slaughterhouse or be tortured for two years before having your throat cut open? I bet you would choose the first option.

Billions of these ill-fated female birds are abused every year for a mere taste and a bad habit. Hens in egg factories have a large portion of their beaks cut off with a burning-hot blade within hours or days of birth. Birds are in pain both during and after the procedure in which no painkillers are used. Chicks, who often have a hard time eating and drinking after their beaks are mutilated, can suffer from hunger and dehydration because their food and water intake are significantly reduced for several weeks after the procedure.

Hens are then shoved into tiny wire "battery" cages, which measure roughly 18 inches by 24 inches and hold up to 10 hens, each of whom has a wingspan up to 36 inches. Even in the best-case scenario, a hen spends its life crowded in a space about the size of a file drawer with several other hens, unable to lift a single wing.

Though hens are typically clean animals, they are so tightly crammed together, that they are forced to urinate and defecate on one another. The stench of ammonia and feces hangs heavy in the air, and disease runs rampant in the filthy, cramped sheds. Many birds die, and survivors are often forced to live with their dying cage mates, who are sometimes left to rot.

The light in the sheds is continuously manipulated to maximize egg production. For two weeks at a time, the hens are fed only reduced-calorie feed. This process induces an extra laying cycle.

Male chicks are worthless to the egg industry, so every year, millions of them are suffocated or thrown into high-speed grinders, called "macerators," while they are still alive.

After about two years in these conditions, the hen's bodies are exhausted, and their egg production drops. These "spent" hens are shipped to slaughterhouses, where their fragile legs are forced into shackles before having their throats cut. By the time they are sent to slaughter, roughly

30 percent of them are suffering from broken bones resulting from neglect, osteoporosis, and rough treatment. Their emaciated bodies are so damaged that their flesh can usually only be turned into chicken soup or for companion-animal food.

Unfortunately, if you care about animal cruelty and the environment, there is no such thing as "I only eat chicken, eggs, or dairy." Whenever an animal is involved in a product be it food or items, there is a terrible price paid by the victims, and we, the consumers, not the slaughterhouses, not the farmers, not the fast-food chains are ultimately responsible for it. Businesses are only responding to customer's demand.

"I love bacon."

Chickens are the most populous breed of farm animal, but in terms of treatment, violence, and psychological abuse, the pig is arguably number one on the list.

Pigs are extraordinarily intelligent. They are curious and insightful animals who are known to be as smart as three-year-old children, and even some primates. Pigs tend to have a lot of similarities with humans in terms of emotions and cognitive faculties, and further scientific research has acknowledged their significant mental capabilities, social nature, and capacity to experience pain, pleasure, fear, and joy. Contrary to popular belief, pigs are naturally hygienic animals and choose remote areas for defecating and urinating far away from their sleeping, living, and feeding areas.

Due to their level of intelligence and emotion, we can only imagine the level of physical and mental torment forced upon them.

Most mother pigs spend their lives in individual "gestation" crates. These crates are about seven feet long and two feet wide too small to allow the animals room to turn around. After giving birth to piglets, sows are moved to "farrowing" crates, which are wide enough for them to lie down and nurse their babies but not big enough for them to stand up or even look at their young.

Piglets are separated from their mothers when they are as young as 10 days old. Once her piglets are gone, the sow is impregnated (raped) again as soon as possible, and the cycle continues for three or four years. When their bodies cannot produce enough for human profit, they are sent to their death. This intensive confinement produces stress and boredom related behavior, such as chewing on cage bars. No criminals, no murderers are treated as severely as these innocent victims.

After they are taken from their mothers, piglets are confined to pens and barns for about six months, fed until they weigh upwards of 280 lbs. and are ready to be sold as meat. Every year in the U.S., millions of male piglets are castrated (usually without being given any painkillers) because consumers supposedly complain of "boar taint" in meat that comes from intact animals.

In incredibly crowded conditions, piglets are prone to stress-related behavior such as cannibalism and tail-biting, so farmers often chop off piglets' tails and use pliers to break off the ends of their teeth, again, without painkillers. For identification purposes, farmers also cut out chunks of the young animals' ears.

These living hell facilities have more in common with concentration camps than what we used to call a farm. Without a trace of natural light, the air is putrid with an intense smell of urine and feces, while worms and flies crawl everywhere.

Infections, bruises, corpses, diseases are omnipresent. There is no comfort, no care, no help, in these prisons when your only purpose in life is to end up on a grocery store shelf.

Transportation

Once pigs reach "market weight," the industry refers to them as "hogs," and they are sent to slaughter. The animals are shipped from all over the U.S. and Canada to slaughterhouses. According to a 2006 industry report, more than one million pigs die on the road to slaughter each year.[4]

Pigs tend to resist getting into the multideck trailers with steep ramps, so workers use sharp electric prods to move them along. These sharp prods not only electrocute the pigs but very often cut open their skin.

Many videos and photos from inside these transport trailers are taken weekly by vegan activists standing in front of

---

[4] https://www.peta.org/issues/animals-used-for-food/animals-used-food-factsheets/pigs-intelligent-animals-suffering-factory-farms-slaughterhouses/

transport trucks entering the slaughterhouse loading area. They show pigs vomiting, trembling, panting, overheating, freezing to death, and all bruised up just to name a few of the horrific conditions they witness.

There is outrage whenever a dog is left in a hot car in the summer. People will smash car windows to rescue a suffocating dog and post about how careless and unacceptable such behavior is. Whoever helps save a dog's life is considered a hero. I support anyone saving animals, but isn't it hypocritical to help one but willingly torture the other? I have seen thermometers showing +40C in trucks packed with farm animals. What about their suffering? What about freezing in those same trucks at -20C in the wintertime? They suffer much longer, often to their death and by the millions. Don't they deserve our outrage and attention too? Are we selfishly turning a blind eye for our love of BBQ ribs?

Slaughterhouses

A typical slaughterhouse kills about 1,000 hogs per hour. The sheer number of animals killed makes it impossible for each pigs' deaths to be humane and painless. Because of improper stunning, many hogs are alive when they reach the scalding-hot water baths, which are intended to soften their skin and remove their hair. The U.S. Department of Agriculture documented humane-slaughter violations at one processing plant, where inspectors found hogs who were walking and squealing after being stunned with a stun gun as many as four times.[5]

Many slaughterhouses use gas chambers to kill hogs. From outside these facilities, you can hear the pigs screaming and gasping in agony as their lungs burn from carbon dioxide. It is nothing short of an animal holocaust. Of all the footage I have seen exposing animal cruelty, gas chambers were among the most unbearable. Can you imagine living it?

How much lower can we stoop as a society? How many more of these sentient beings must die before we come to our senses? This is all futile: a nightmare we could easily avoid. We don't need bacon or ham to survive, yet we are taking billions of innocent lives, destroying the environment, and damaging our health. Factory farming needs to be outlawed, period.

Dairy, a Cruel Business

When I was a teenager, I worked in dairy farms as a cattle hoof claw trimmer. Cattle are chained to the same position for most of the day, due to overgrowth, their claws can become sensitive and prone to lameness. Their back claws often rot and get infected with worms from standing in feces and urine for long periods of time.

My job consisted of taking the cows one by one into a mobile cage to trim their claws, treat lameness, sole ulcers, or lesions. The first step was to strap the cow's head tight to the sidebar of the cage so the cow would not move

---

[5] https://www.peta.org/issues/animals-used-for-food/animals-used-food-factsheets/pigs-intelligent-animals-suffering-factory-farms-slaughterhouses/

violently and hurt herself in the process.

We would then isolate her leg and strap her hoof through a manual gear that we would turn to bring the sole facing upward. We would then trim her claw using an electric buffer, the same kind used for home renovations. Very often, when coming across an infection, a lesion, an ulcer or white worms, depending on the severity, we would buff her hoof until we reached the "clean" non-infected area.

In other words, we would buff until we could see the red, fleshy part of her hoof. Without ever given anesthesia, or any form of painkillers, the cows would panic and scream in agony. I remember seeing their big eyeballs rolling backwards while saliva dribbled from their mouths. Once the job was over, we would spray disinfectant to the open wound, wrap it with bandages, and free the cow. Immediately after, the cow could hardly stand on that leg and would often fall flat on the floor. We would use electric prods to get them standing and pull them back into their pen as fast as possible.

We worked on dozens of cows per day, and many dairy farms per week. It was a gruesome business, one that I learned to accept as "normal". I wasn't a bad guy, but social proof (as I mentioned earlier), made me blind to the suffering that I was inflicting on the "livestock". I wasn't making the connection between the animal and my contribution to its misery.

If anyone would have been caught doing this to a dog or cat, he would have been charged with animal cruelty. What gives us the right to treat farm animals with so much violence? How are we separating them from our pets or wild species we vouch to protect?

"In fact, if one person is unkind to an animal it is considered to be cruelty, but where a lot of people are unkind to animals, especially in the name of commerce, the cruelty is condoned and, once large sums of money are at stake, will be defended to the last by otherwise intelligent people."

Ruth Harrison

"I love cheese so much I could never give it up."

People often ask me what is wrong with milk or cheese since, unlike meat, we are not killing the cows. Well, not only are we killing the dairy cow after only four or five years, but we also slay each of their calves to drink or use what is rightfully theirs.[6]

Given the chance, cows nurture their young and form lifelong friendships with one another. They play games and have a wide range of emotions and personality traits. But most cows raised for the dairy industry are intensively confined, leaving them unable to fulfill their most basic desires, such as nursing their calves, even for a single day. Instead they are treated like machines, genetically manipulated and pumped full of antibiotics and hormones to increase milk production. While cows suffer on factory farms, humans who drink their milk increase their chances

---

[6] https://www.sciencedaily.com/releases/2015/04/150428081801.htm (2015)

of developing heart disease, diabetes, cancer, and many other ailments.

Cows produce milk for the same reason that humans do; to nourish their young. But calves on dairy farms are taken away from their mothers when they are just a day old. They are fed milk replacers (including cattle blood) so that their mothers' milk can be sold to humans. The calves are then sent to the slaughterhouse to be sold as veal.

Female cows are artificially inseminated, or in other words, raped, shortly after their first birthday. After giving birth, they lactate for 10 months and are inseminated again, continuing the cycle. Some spend their entire lives standing on concrete floors while others are confined to massive, crowded lots, where they are forced to live amid their own feces. A North Carolina dairy farm exposed following revelations from a whistleblower that the cows were forced to eat, walk and sleep in knee-deep waste.[7]

Cows have a natural lifespan of about 20 years and can produce milk for eight or nine years. However, the stress caused by the conditions on factory farms leads to disease, lameness, and reproductive problems that render cows worthless to the dairy industry by the time that they're four or five years old, at which time they are sent to be slaughtered.

On any given day, there are more than nine million cows on U.S. dairy farms, about 12 million fewer than there were in 1950. Yet milk production has continued to increase from

---

[7] https://www.independent.ie/ca/videos/world-news/shocking-video-footage-of-cows-forced-to-stand-in-kneedeep-manure-for-hours-30513272.html

116 billion pounds of milk per year in 1950 to 215 billion pounds in 2017. Typically, these animals would produce only enough milk to meet the needs of their calves, but genetic manipulation and, in some cases, antibiotics and hormones are used to cause each cow to produce more than 23,000 pounds of milk each year.[8] Cows are also fed unnatural, high-protein diets, which can include chicken feathers and fish because their natural diet of grass would not provide the nutrients that they need to produce such massive amounts of milk.

If any dog breeding facilities were treating their animals this way, it would be shut down immediately. Again, what have farmed animals done to be ignored and mistreated in such a way?

We can comfortably live without cheese and milk. There are dozens of delicious, nutritious plant-based milks like almond, oat, rice, cashew or coconut milk. New cheese alternatives are coming out every week and are more delicious than ever. I once fooled my French stepfather with a non-dairy goat cheese, and he never realized the difference.

We just covered the treatment of chicken, pigs, and cows but we could go on with the spine-chilling treatment of geese for foie gras, the awful life of sheep abused for their wool, or the hideous business of thanksgiving turkey. The list is as long as the animal products on your grocer's shelves. Remember, every time you buy an animal product,

---

[8] https://qz.com/1649587/the-way-we-breed-cows-is-setting-them-up-for-extinction/ (2019)

be it food or by-products the real price is paid by the animal forced to give up its life for it. There is no way of avoiding it, dog lovers don't eat dogs, animal lovers don't eat animals.

Entertainment and forced labor

Circuses, zoos, aquariums, elephant riding, horse racing, and horse carriages are all using against their will for human entertainment or labor. People consider these practices to be acceptable, but are they?

The use of elephants for tourism has become regrettably trendy. Vacations boasting elephant rides or contact with pachyderms have popped up across Asia. Many Instagrammers proudly pose with elephants thinking it's cool and exotic, but while these might appear to be fun activities for you, the reality is that the experience is anything but amusing for the elephants.

Although elephants are incredibly intelligent and docile by nature, none of the behaviors, tricks, or forced labor exhibited by captive elephants in the tourism industry are natural. One may question how an elephant of a few tons could be so submissive to a human of a few dozen kilos? Why would such a powerful animal not just walk away?

In a natural context they would, but to get these wild animals to obey their masters, they must undergo an extraordinarily cruel breaking process, called "Phajaan".[9] The Phajaan program aims to break the elephant's spirit.

---

[9] https://theecologist.org/2018/aug/20/tourism-and-torture-our-sublime-elephants

24

Baby elephants between three to six years old are kept in small crates like those found in the pig farming industry. With their feet tied with ropes, and their limbs stretched, these helpless victims are repeatedly beaten with sharp sticks, continuously screamed at, and starved of food. Bull hooks (a tool used in most forms of elephant control) will be used to stab the head, slash the skin, and tug the ears.

The Phajaan may last for weeks, and the babies have no rest from physical and mental torture. Gradually, their spirit will break, they stop fighting back, and their handlers achieve control. Only then, when the animal has learned it cannot resist humans can you possibly ride an elephant's back and take an Instagram selfie.

Horse Carriages

Ever enjoyed a horse carriage ride? Do you have them in your city? They are all over the world, and at first sight, everything about them seems ordinary. From the animal's perspective though, it is nothing short of slavery. If you look from a different angle, you will see a sad horse, strapped to a carriage, metal guides in his mouth, eye blinds and all sort of straps meant to control it. He has no choice, either he executes his human orders, or he gets beaten. Worse, if he refuses to submit and work, he will be sent to a slaughterhouse and sold as cheap minced meat. What choice do they have?

Horses are highly social herd animals who prefer living in groups. They are meant to roam free and enjoy independence just like we do. What right do we have to force them to pull heavy carriages through traffic, pollution, and noise, on a burning summer day or cold winter night?

There is nothing romantic or fun in abusing another sentient being for our selfish pleasure.

There are many other ways to discover a city. For the horse, your joy ride equals a life of confinement, loneliness, and suffering. Please avoid them and help end this cruel practice and any other form of animal exploitation.

4. HUMAN ANATOMY

"Man was not born to be a carnivore."

Albert Einstein

Almost every time I discuss veganism with other people, they tell me that humans are carnivores or omnivores, and that eating meat is not only natural, but necessary. Though widely believed, these are general misconceptions. Let's explore this further.

Meat eaters will be disappointed to hear that from a biological point of view, we have almost nothing in common with carnivores or omnivores.

When referring to humans, I would rather use the term *cheating* omnivore because of our need to cook fresh meat in order to digest it. Tartare and sushi may be an exception, though the former and the latter must be selected from a very specific part of the animal and eaten extremely fresh. But even so, many people still end up with food poisoning from eating these dishes.

Could you eat raw chicken? A raw pig? Could you eat a carcass? Have you ever witnessed carnivorous or omnivorous animals having a BBQ in the wild?

The truth is, most of our anatomy is comparable to herbivores. We cannot swallow chunks of food like dogs, we grind and chew while we eat, like herbivores. Humans have no natural skills to catch prey. We have no claws on our hands or feet, a trademark of carnivores and omnivores. Our mouth-to-head opening ratio is considerably smaller than carnivores and omnivores which allows them to bite and kill their prey. Our teeth are short and flat, just like those of herbivores. Despite popular belief, our tiny "canine teeth" are of no use to kill an animal.

Could a human chase a deer, capture it, bite it to death, and then eat it whole? The fur, eyes, paws, blood, and organs? If you place a living guinea pig and a carrot in a crib with a hungry child, would the child instinctively kill and eat the rodent or go for the carrot?

Humans require dietary fiber to maintain regular bowel functioning. Carnivores and omnivores do not. A human's gastrointestinal tract is more similar in length to that of an herbivore's than it is to that of a carnivore or omnivore.[10] Carnivores and omnivores thrive on fat and animal protein, while the same diet will create diseases and other health problems in humans.

A diet rich in fat and animal protein is linked to heart disease, a leading cause of death in the United States.[11]

According to Dr. Kim Williams, former president of the American College of Cardiology, no one should adopt the

---

[10] https://www.vivahealth.org.uk/wheat-eaters-or-meat-eaters/length-digestive-tract

[11] https://stacks.cdc.gov/view/cdc/60902

infamous ketogenic diet (mainly fat and animal protein) over the long term unless weight loss is more important than lifespan.

Our anatomy and nature are one of plant-based eaters. Let's take our heads out of the sand, we are not carnivores or omnivores. Arguing otherwise would be based on myths, not common sense and facts.

5.   ANIMAL PROTEIN & HEALTH

In this chapter, we are going to discuss the different health impacts associated with eating non-vegan food. Most of us are eating animal products without questioning its effects on our health.

After all, everybody is doing it, and the food industry is still organized largely around animal consumption. Many intelligent, compassionate, and educated people believe eating animals is something that we must do to maintain our health and vitality.

Fortunately, science is now on our side. The most recent studies confirm that the optimal diet for nutrition and health is one where we get all our nutrients from plant-based foods like vegetables, fruits, grains, legumes, seeds, and nuts.

Protein

People worry a lot about protein specifically, so let's learn more about what proteins are and the implications of eating animal protein. First, it is important to know that protein is abundant both in plant foods as well as in animal foods. Proteins are abundant in meat, fish, dairy, and eggs as well as in grains, legumes, seeds, and nuts.

But what exactly are proteins? Proteins are chains of organic compounds called amino acids which are joined together by peptide bonds. The term essential amino acid refers to nine amino acids that our bodies cannot synthesize, and we, therefore, need to get from food. These nine are: leucine, isoleucine, lysine, tryptophan, histidine, phenylalanine, valine, methionine and threonine.

Most proteins found in animal-based foods contain the nine essential amino acids our body requires, thus why people refer to animal proteins as "complete". Plant proteins, on the other hand, with some exceptions like soy, quinoa, seitan, and buckwheat which are complete proteins, are individually lacking some of the nine essential amino acids. That's where the trap is and where most people get confused thinking plant-based proteins are not good enough.

It is true that most plant-based proteins are lacking some essential amino acids if taken separately but, combining different veggies, nuts, grains or beans together, will give you all the essential amino acids you need and much more nutrients than animal-based proteins. This is what we call "complementing". Some good examples are mixing rice and beans, hummus and pita bread, a peanut butter sandwich on whole grain toast, cereal with almond milk, or lentil and vegetable soup. If you eat a balanced and varied vegan diet, you will have a plentiful supply of the nine essential amino acids, and it is not necessary to eat them all within the same meal. You are probably already complementing your meals without even thinking about it.

When we eat proteins, whether beef or nuts, the proteins that we eat do not go straight to our muscles and begin to function in our body. The proteins are first broken down in our digestive system to their simplest element. We then synthesize proteins according to our needs. If we're going to synthesize muscle or if we're going to synthesize an enzyme, our body could not care less whether the given amino acids came from a plant or an animal because they are identical. In ourselves, in our DNA, we have the recipes to rebuild the proteins suiting our specific needs.

Animal proteins are built up into a complex array of protein strains your body needs to break down into separate amino acids before using them. This significantly slows down digestion and forces your body to work harder than it needs to. Green vegetables such as broccoli or lentils, for example, are rich in easily absorbed amino acids.

When you fuel yourself with foods that are easier to digest, your body can direct more energy into healing the wear-and-tear on your muscles caused by a workout. Not only will you heal quicker on a diet of plant proteins that often has more nutrients than meat, you will also have more energy for the next day's work out.

Plants can provide you with all the proteins you need. Just look at some of the biggest and strongest animals on Earth: elephants, rhinoceros, bulls, horses, and gorillas are all herbivores.

Cholesterol

Animal proteins, unlike plant-based foods, are packaged with bad cholesterol. Our liver synthesizes good cholesterol for all our bodily functions, we don't need to get it from external sources.

People eat foods like chicken and turkey because they are white meat or because they're "lean meat". They think that eating them baked, boiled, or grilled, would make them a healthy meal.

But unfortunately, regardless of the way it is cooked, animal flesh has a high cholesterol content which can end up getting burrowed in the lining of our arteries. This build-up can cause atherosclerosis, or cardiovascular diseases.

The only source of cholesterol in the world apart from what your body produces, is animal and animal-derived products. All plant-based foods are entirely cholesterol-free.

Fiber

Unlike plant protein, which comes packed with fiber, antioxidants, and phytonutrients, animal protein comes with none of the preceding. Meat, eggs, poultry, dairy, fish, and other animal foods have no fiber whatsoever.

In an effort to get enough protein, many people tend to eat large amounts of animal foods, which displaces plant foods that have essential nutrients. Fiber deficiencies are far more common than not.

For example, The Institute of Medicine recommends that men consume 38 grams of fiber, but the average adult only eats about 15 grams per day, less than half the recommended amount.[12] In fact, according to the USDA, almost all Americans, 95%, do not get an adequate amount of dietary fiber.

High fiber intake is associated with decreased cancer risk, specifically colon and breast cancers, as well as a lower risk of ulcerative colitis, Crohn's disease, constipation, and diverticulitis. It may also reduce the risk of stroke, high cholesterol, and heart disease.[13]

Dairy

Is milk good or bad for you? Years of lobbying and marketing campaigns funded by the dairy industry to influence both the public and governments, has elevated milk into an almost supernatural liquid essential to our bones and development.

At the same time, in recent years, several studies have also associated milk with an increased risk of oncology and immune-related pathologies like multiple sclerosis and diabetes. So, who should we believe?

Most of us are not doctors or scientists to analyze those reports, and I certainly would not want to get deeper into a subject I'm not qualified for. There is one good argument though that could help us all see clearly through the contradictions in those claims: The 2019 Canadian Food

---

[12] https://www.ncbi.nlm.nih.gov/pmc/articles/PMC6124841/
Closing America's Fiber Intake Gap 2016

[13] https://www.ncbi.nlm.nih.gov/pmc/articles/PMC6315720/
Whole Fruits and Fruit Fiber Emerging Health Effects 2018

Guide.[14]

Dr. Hasan Hutchinson, director-general of Health Canada's office of nutrition policy and promotion says the day before the guide was made public:

"We were very clear that when we were looking at the evidence base that we were not going to be using reports that have been funded by industry as well."

Interestingly, something is noticeably missing from the guide: a daily dose of dairy! Health Canada's new 2019 food guide drops its former "milk and alternatives" food group altogether. As you can imagine, the changes have been praised by advocates for plant-based diets but have raised the ire of the dairy lobby.

Animals produce milk specifically for their own species offspring. Each mother's milk has its own levels of protein, carbohydrates, fat, minerals, vitamins, and hormones. The milk of a cow, a pig, a porcupine or a rat are differently balanced to suit each species biological needs. Humans have no business drinking the milk of another animal.

From an evolutionary point of view, milk is a strange food for an adult human. Until 10,000 years ago we didn't domesticate animals and weren't able to drink milk.

Most humans naturally stop producing significant amounts of lactase, the enzyme needed to properly metabolize lactose, (the sugar in milk), sometime between the ages of two and five. In fact, for most mammals, the prevailing

---

[14] https://food-guide.canada.ca/en/

condition is to stop producing the enzymes needed to digest and metabolize milk after they have been weaned.

Our bodies just weren't made to digest milk regularly. Instead, most scientists now agree that it's better for us to get calcium, potassium, protein, and fats from other food sources, like vegetables, fruits, beans, whole grains, nuts, seeds, and seaweed.

Delicious and healthy alternatives like almond, oat, rice, or soy milk are now widely available in grocery stores to replace cruel, polluting, health-hazardous cow milk. The choice to make is self-evident.

Fish

We'll dig deeper into the subject in a later chapter, but I want to point something out about fish. Fish are animals too, not swimming vegetables with eyes. Fish is an animal protein associated with complications previously mentioned in this chapter, including cholesterol and toxic mercury concentration. Fish is not a sustainable alternative to meat.

Cancer and Animal Proteins

A study from the University of Southern California draws links between animal proteins and cancer.

> "That chicken wing you're eating could be as deadly as a cigarette. In a new study that tracked a large sample of adults for nearly two decades, researchers have found that eating a diet rich in animal proteins

during middle age makes you four times more likely to die of cancer than someone with a low-protein diet, a mortality risk factor comparable to smoking. 'There's a misconception that because we all eat, understanding nutrition is simple. But the question is not whether a certain diet allows you to do well for three days, but can it help you survive to be 100?' Said Valter Longo PhD, Professor of Biogerontology at the USC Davis School of Gerontology and director of the USC Longevity Institute."[15]

If you have your health at heart, I strongly suggest reading this full study online. The study determines a direct link between high protein consumption and cancer mortality. Middle-aged people who eat lots of animal protein including meat, milk, and cheese are also more susceptible to early death in general.

People eating a high-protein diet were also 74 percent more likely to die of any cause, including diabetes, within the study period compared to those who ate a low-protein diet.

The Real "High Quality" Food

Given all the issues, the so-called "high quality" aspect of animal protein might be more appropriately described as "high risk" according to Sofia Ochoa M.D.

There is no need to worry about protein adequacy if you are eating a well-rounded diet of plant foods like vegetables,

---

[15] https://www.sciencedaily.com/releases/2014/03/140304125639.htm

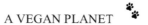

fruits, legumes, grains, nuts, and seeds.

Dr. Walter Willett, the chair of Harvard's Department of Nutrition:

"To the metabolic systems engaged in protein production and repair, it is immaterial whether amino acids come from animal or plant protein. However, protein is not consumed in isolation. Instead, it is packaged with a host of other nutrients. I, therefore, recommend that you pick the best protein packages by emphasizing plant sources of protein rather than animal sources."

I hope you now understand a little better why plant-based nutrients are the real "high quality" foods we should find on our plate for optimal health. We should also remind ourselves, that no matter how bad eating meat, fish or dairy may be to us, no matter how devastating it may be for the environment, the real price of our food choices is paid by the animals.

6. A BALANCED VEGAN DIET

"Give me six hours to chop down a tree, and I will spend the first four sharpening the ax."

Abraham Lincoln

Preparation is key to any successful endeavor. Learning the basics and planning will significantly increase your chances of implementing a new habit in your life. If you do not have a clear and defined "why" for the efforts you are putting into achieving a goal, the first challenges you face may derail you from your objective and set you back on old habits.

If you have never been to a gym before, it is unlikely you will come out with the right training program without first getting tips from a coach. You may get discouraged for not losing weight or gaining muscles and start believing a fit body is not for you.

If the first time you play golf you try to drive 300 yards with a putter club, you may think you are terrible at this sport when in fact, you simply didn't know how to use a golf set properly.

Many people have tried a vegan diet only to give up within a few weeks or months. Lack of energy, not knowing what to eat, missing bacon, missing cheese, peer pressure at the BBQ, are all common excuses to get back to meat-eating. If you are careless with your preparation, like anything else, you are severely limiting your chances of success.

Taking on a new diet means acting three times daily, it could be quite different from what you are accustomed to. It's not difficult or complicated, but you will need to build new habits, get a little bit of food knowledge, experiment with new recipes, and remind yourself the morality behind your decision to avoid that juicy steak at the restaurant.

The fact that society is still mainly non-vegan adds a challenge as the food supply still orbits around animal-based products. Do not worry, you will quickly adapt and find what you need. With the multiplication of vegan products and alternatives, there has never been an easier time to go vegan.

As a new vegan, it would not be wise to simply cut off all animal-based products for lettuce, carrots, and tofu. Such a diet would obviously lead to nutrient deficiencies. In this case, the vegan diet would not be to blame, but rather the lack of knowledge in balancing nutrient intake. It seems obvious, but it is essential when going vegan, to replace animal-based products instead of just removing them from the food you eat.

The vegan version of a chicken caesar salad is not simply a salad without chicken, bacon bits, parmesan or creamy dressing. Rather, it is a salad with roasted almonds in replacement of the chicken, smoky coconut flakes in replacement of bacon, plant-based parmesan, and a delicious cashew-based dressing. This way, it will be full of nutrients you need, and it will taste just as good (or better) than the original version.

Misunderstandings lead people to criticize veganism. Most hospital patients are non-vegans who are being treated for proven food-related chronic diseases. But as they are the population's majority, very few will point the food as being the root cause of their conditions. Making the connection would mean having to change their own food habits. It is easier to blame genes, external factors or plain bad luck.

On the other side, being the minority, if a vegan has any health issues, a cold, lower energy or weight loss, many people will single out the vegan diet as being the culprit. It is a defensive mechanism that many non-vegans use to comfort themselves in their choices, often unconsciously.

If you want to learn more about nutrients, I invite you to read the chapter Nutrients at the end of this book.

7. MY PERSONAL EXPERIENCE

"I always say that eating a plant-based diet is the secret weapon of enhanced athletic performance."

Rich Roll
Named one of the 25 fittest men in the world by Fitness Magazine 2009.

On a personal level, I first became vegan over 20 years ago. I would by now be suffering from malnutrition issues if plant-based food was lacking in nutrients. I take my physical fitness level very seriously. I am 185 pounds and six feet tall. I have never had a broken bone or suffered from any illnesses. I work out at the gym daily, and I run, swim, bike, and climb in my spare time.

In the fall of 2018, I ran my first marathon with two months' notice finishing under four hours. Wanting to explore my mental and physical capabilities further, I registered for my first extreme triathlon, the Xtri World Tour Triathlon Canadaman challenge. This extreme triathlon combines 3.8km of swimming, 180km of biking, 42.2km marathon with a 4km elevation gain. With no previous biking or freestyle swimming experience, I only had 6 months to learn these two disciplines. I managed to finish the race within 16 hours and 32 minutes, ranking 95th out of 190 participants coming from 20 different countries.

My energy level remained stable throughout, I didn't suffer any injuries or joint/muscle pain. I fully recovered just two days after the race and went back to training the same week.

Three weeks later, I participated in the crossing of Lake Tremblant, a twelve-kilometer-long swimming marathon. I exceeded the time limit set for the race 800 meters from the finish line but still, I swam the course in five hours and 30 minutes. This crossing amounted to three times my longest distance swam in open water.

I took these challenges for two reasons. First, I wanted to learn more about myself, and second I wanted to debunk the myth about animal protein being essential to sport performance. Leading by example was important to me.

As an entrepreneur, I live a hectic and sometimes stressful life. I sleep an average of six hours per night but still have all the energy I need to go about my busy schedule. Though many other factors contribute to my well-being, like regular exercise, adequate sleep, and a positive attitude, overall, there is no doubt a vegan diet has been fundamental to my health and fitness.

8. VEGETARIAN

When thinking about the environment and animal issues, many take the steps of becoming a vegetarian. This usually means not eating animal flesh but fish, dairy and eggs. I would most definitely applaud anyone taking a step in the right direction but is it sustainable? I have discussed the dairy and egg issues in previous chapters, but what about fish?

The oceans are already tremendously overfished and all signals from the scientific community point towards a massive decline in fish stock within a decade or two. If tomorrow everyone started relying on fish or seafood for their proteins, we would simply collapse the ocean's ecosystems within years.

The U.N. warns that 90% of our world's fish stock is at or near unsustainable levels.[16] Nearly one-third of all species of fish have declined in population in the last 15 years, and many species may be wiped out in the next decade.

This decline in fish populations is leading to increasing conflicts between fishers and wildlife who eat fish to survive.

---

[16] http://www.fao.org/3/a-i5555e.pdf

Some fishermen intentionally kill or maim seals, birds, and marine mammals whom they perceive as a threat to their catch.

Peta also reported the following:

> "Many species are in decline as a result of fishing. The number of Steller's sea lions in the Bering Sea has declined by 80 percent since the 1950s. An estimated 100,000 seals, whales, and porpoises and a million birds every year become entangled in nets and drown. Because dolphins habitually swim with schools of tuna, the tuna fishing industry even today "accidentally" drowns at least 20,000 of these intelligent mammals annually. Critically endangered sea turtles have been killed incidentally by the thousands by shrimp trawlers. The fact is, eating one fish result in the deaths of many."[17]

It was pretty heartbreaking to look at a video of a commercial fishing boat mechanically hoarding onboard its massive net of thousands of suffocating fish. But what made it even more dramatic was seeing orcas swimming around the boat looking at their only sources of food being stolen by humans, a land animal. Imagine if whales invaded a farmer's corn field and began swallowing up most of the crops. What a nightmare that would be for a family and community that relies on this source of food for survival.

On top of dealing with these destructive fishing practices, ocean inhabitants are also faced with the threat of plastic

---

[17] https://www.peta.org/about-peta/faq/what-about-fish-in-the-wild-caught-by-commercial-fishers/

pollution. Millions of fish, sea mammals and birds are dying each year from plastic obstructing their digestive systems. Warming water temperatures, and ocean acidification further burden an already weakened ocean ecosystem. A vegetarian diet is simply unsustainable to feed seven billion humans.

What about Fish Farming?

Salmon, one of the most popular fish on the market is now factory farmed at 70%.[18] One would think fish farming would relieve some pressure off the wild fish stock but unfortunately it is not that simple. Given that salmon are carnivorous, it can take up to five kilos of fish meal to yield one kilo of salmon flesh. By eating fish that eats fish, we are simply taking away pressure from one species to put more on many others. Plus, farmed salmon are sometimes able to escape from their polluting oceanside pens they are raised in, spreading disease or undesirable genes to wild populations. On top of the intensive use of antibiotics, fish feed has also been shown to have been contaminated with toxins that can make their way into the food supply.

As a society, we have created a massive problem by overpopulating the Earth without ever considering the consequences. With almost eight billion mouths to feed, even the vastness of the oceans and their fish stock is not enough. The only way out, as of today, is for the world to go plant-based and fast.

Going vegetarian will only displace one problem to another.

---

[18] https://www.worldwildlife.org/industries/farmed-salmon

At this time in our history, we must all come together and make this communal effort. It is not an option, it is no longer a personal choice, it is a matter of survival and the only chance we have to offer our children a decent planet to live on.

9. ENVIRONMENTAL COST & GLOBAL WARMING

"The demand for meat has a multiplier effect of 10. You need ten times as much land, ten times as much feed, ten times as much water to produce one calorie of meat as you do to have one calorie of vegetables or grain."

Mr. Peter Brabeck-Letmathe, Chairman of Nestlé

Global warming, which is caused by greenhouse gas emissions, is one of the defining issues of our time. Keeping temperature increase below the two degrees Celsius mark should be one of humanity's utmost priority.

Failing at this objective will result in catastrophic consequences such as melting glaciers, rising sea levels, disrupted ocean current patterns, cataclysmic storms, extreme drought, and temperature changes all of which will make life on Earth a living nightmare.[19]

With ever-changing weather conditions within a declining ecosystem, agriculture would be under tremendous pressure to keep producing enough food for everyone. All these factors combined could easily lead to a massive economic crisis, dooming humanity.

[19] www.un.org/en/climatechange/reports.shtml

Scientists agree that we only have a few years left to take massive action before climate change becomes irreversible. How could we possibly explain ourselves to future generations knowing our inaction and unaccountability has darkened their future? Never in the history of humanity has a generation had so much responsibility on their shoulders. Now the question is: how are we going to respond to it?

We could sometimes feel powerless and point the finger at big corporations or governments, but let's not forget, they are merely a reflection of ourselves. We want our politicians to take serious action but, as individuals, are we leading by example? We can point at Coca Cola for manufacturing billions of plastic bottles that end up in the oceans, but who buys them? How often do we go to Starbucks and ask for a latte in a takeaway cup with a plastic lid only to throw it away 30 min later? We may recycle but recycled or not; plastic stays on Earth for 400 years!

As consumers and voters, we have enormous power. Multinational businesses would go bankrupt within months if we stop buying their products. They cannot force you to buy their bottled water, it's called purchase power; you decide not them. The products you see on the retailer's shelves mirrors the consumer's demand.

The latter applies to politicians as well. They are ready to do almost anything to get elected. They regularly scrutinize their electing bases doing internal surveys to come out with platforms that could win them votes. If they realize the environment is their voter's number one priority, they will fight each other to come out with the best solutions to win votes.

Some may say we already want less pollution and less global warming but, do we? Recycling, which means throwing plastic in a different bin and cutting our use of straws in cocktails is hardly going to make any difference. And by the way, not using plastic straws to help sea life but eating fish for dinner, is quite a paradox.

What I mean here is we must do a little more than the minimum effort. Fighting global warming and the destruction of our ecosystems do not require us to go to war but merely changing some of our daily habits. It is not enough to read about it and wish for a change; we must act.

"I don't want your hope. I don't want you to be hopeful. I want you to panic... To act as if the house was on fire, because it is"

Greta Thunberg 15-year-old environmental activist

Did you know that palm oil causes deforestation, and the extinction of orangutans? One simple way we can help is boycotting palm oil. By law, ingredients are listed on food labels. Get into the habit of reading them before you buy and learn about food products that are better for the environment. Swapping your favorite chocolate spread like Nutella for another brand, is a small price to pay to help our planet. You keep eating delicious chocolate spread; you only pick a more sustainable one. After a while, you will have reorganized your shopping list, and you won't even think about it anymore. Organic, local products, non-processed or natural ingredients are often useful clues as to know if a product is a better choice.

If you're like me and you are fed up with the billions of disposable coffee cups wasted every year, I recommend bringing your own mug or thermos to Starbucks. Keep your thermos or reusable cup with you at work, in your car, or your handbag. It's a simple habit to develop, and many coffee shops will reward you by offering a rebate.

"What difference will one disposable cup make?" is a thought we should avoid. If seven billion people think this way, seven billion more cups will forever be in the environment. Multiplied by 365 days a year, that's over 2.5 trillion cups wasted. focusing on our daily actions, and doing what is right, we become leaders and encourage others to follow in our steps.

"If everyone ate vegan, food-related carbon emissions would fall by 70%"

Greenpeace

Plastic reduction, recycling, public transport, local organic food, eco-friendly purchases, green voting are all impactful actions each of us can easily do to help the situation. But did you know, the most significant impact a human can have towards global warming and the destruction of our ecosystem is going vegan?

That may be surprising, but researchers at the University of Oxford found that cutting meat and dairy products from your diet could reduce an individual's carbon footprint from food by up to 73 percent.[20]

Meanwhile, if everyone stopped eating these foods, they found that global farmland use would reduce by 75 percent, an area equivalent to the size of the US, China, Australia, and the EU combined.

Not only would this result in a massive drop in greenhouse gas emissions, it would also free up wild land lost to agriculture, which is one of the primary causes of mass wildlife extinction.

"A vegan diet is probably the single biggest way to reduce your impact on planet Earth, not just greenhouse gases, but global acidification, eutrophication, land use, and water use," said Joseph Poore, at the University of Oxford, UK, who led the research. "It is far bigger than cutting down on your flights or buying an electric car," he said, as these only cut greenhouse gas emissions.

Currently, there are over seven billion people on the face of our planet, predicted to hit the nine billion mark by 2050. Arable land is covering approximately eight billion acres of the Earth's surface, the equivalent of about six billion football fields.

Did you know it requires the equivalent of two football fields of Arable land per person per year to produce the Standard American Diet (SAD) which is heavily comprised of animal protein and dairy? If all seven billion of us were consuming the SAD, we would need more than two planet

---

[20] http://www.ox.ac.uk/news/2018-06-01-new-estimates-environmental-cost-food

Earths to feed us all. Unfortunately, we only have one.[21]

On the same amount of land that it requires to feed one person the SAD, you can feed 14 people the vegan diet. If everyone in the world consumed a whole food, plant-based diet, we could save nearly five out of six billion football fields worth of arable land. This is 83% of arable land that could be returned to forested area to regenerate the lungs of the planet or to expand food production to meet the needs of a growing world population.

"Be the change you want to see in the world."

Ghandi

The production of livestock has pushed the use of monocultures, extensive use of pesticide, fertilizer and the development of GMO crops which are all destroying bio diversification, polluting rivers, oceans and earth is topsoil.

Add precious drinking water, transportation, transformation, and conservation of the meat, and it all becomes very clear why a vegan diet is so vital for our planet and its seven billion inhabitants.

Did you know the production of one kilo of beef uses 15,000 liters of water?[22] That's the equivalent of approximately 100 showers for a single burger!

---

[21] https://www.ncbi.nlm.nih.gov/pmc/articles/PMC5899434/
[22] http://web.unep.org/environmentassembly/15000-litres-water-produce-1-kilo-beef

If we are serious about the environment and global warming, let's act today and adopt a plant-based way of life.

10. A VEGAN ECONOMY

According to Dr. Marco Springmann of Oxford University, not only would veganism result in a healthier planet, it would be a wealthier one too.

"If the world adopted a vegan diet in the year 2050, in that single year it could cut greenhouse gas emissions by two thirds, save $1.5trillion in climate damages and healthcare-related expenditure, and reduce global mortality by 10 per cent, which means eight fewer million deaths from chronic diseases" said Dr. Springmann.[23]

This interesting and thorough study highlighted a direct link between health, environmental, and economic benefits deriving from the adoption of a vegan diet.

Healthcare is by far the most significant expenditure of all developed countries.[24] To put things into perspective, military expenses account for less than 20% of all healthcare budgets of the G7 countries, (US, Canada, UK, France, Italy, Germany, Japan) respectively.

The U.S. spends about 18% of their Gross Domestic Product (GDP) on healthcare compared to the other G7 nations who spend about 10%. Military expenditure on the

---

[23] http://www.oxfordtoday.ox.ac.uk/interviews/what-if-we-all-turned-vegan-2050
[24] https://data.worldbank.org/indicator/SH.XPD.GHED.GE.ZS

other hand, accounts for only 1.2% to 3.5% of these countries' GDPs.

Americans spent a massive 650 billion dollars on their military in 2018 (3.47% of GDP).[25] But a new analysis from U.S. federal government actuaries say that Americans spent a staggering $3.5 trillion on health care in 2018, or (18% of GDP). Even at 650 billion in military spending a year, this only represents 18% of the health care cost.[26]

The all-important education spending average only 5% of GDP for most developed countries.[27] The health care's budget still takes the lion's share of most government's budget, even when combining education and military spending.

It is then clear that any improvement of a nation's health would results in impactful economic gains for almost any country. Billions of dollars a year could be redirected to education, which, in an ideal world, should be the most funded of all budgets. How many educational, environmental, or social projects could receive funding with those savings? No tax raise, no spending cuts. All of these benefits are within reach with a few simple changes in our diet.

On an individual level, how much more money could each of us save on prescription drugs, medical equipment,

---

[25] https://data.worldbank.org/indicator/MS.MIL.XPND.CD

[26] https://www.cms.gov/research-statistics-data-and-systems/statistics-trends-and-reports/nationalhealthexpenddata/nationalhealthaccountshistorical.html

[27] https://data.worldbank.org/indicator/SE.XPD.TOTL.GD.ZS

insurance costs, or loss of revenue due to illness?

Less pollution due to animal agriculture would mean cleaner air, land, lakes, and rivers enhancing our quality of life. Coupled with other factors, this could rank a nation's standards of living higher amongst developed countries and attract more investments.

The financial advantages of a cleaner environment do not stop there. Extra money is needed to treat polluted water before it can be used to drink. Cottage properties are less valuable when they sit on lakes that are thick with algae. Penthouse condos with views clouded by smog are worth less than those with unobstructed vistas. Farmland falls in value when crops are harder to grow because of air, soil, or water pollution.

More research is needed to fill the gaps in our understanding of pollution's costs, but it's clear it has a significant impact on our economy.

Jobs

Some could rightfully question the impact on agriculture and food transformation jobs within a vegan society. In the short term, it is inevitable that many positions would be lost in the slaughterhouses and factory farm businesses but let's not forget people won't stop eating, they will simply eat different food.

When petrol became the number one fossil fuel in the early 20th century, the coal industry started to decline along with its workforce, but it created more jobs in the oil sector. The same applies to electric cars today. This new technology may hit regular thermal engines car manufacturers, but as the job market is highly adaptable, more positions will be created along with the electrification's development. For example, Tesla, an electric car company, now employs over 45,000 workers.

Beyond Meat, the first public company to mass-produce vegan burgers and other plant-based meats created hundreds of jobs and is now massively expanding due to an almost limitless market. The food transformation industry would adapt and manufacture vegan products, while farmers would follow suit to supply the new demand.

Certainly, this will require some adaptation, but it will also create numerous business opportunities transforming an old animal product-based system into a new sustainable plant-based one.

Changes, evolution, and new technologies are driving factors of economic growth. We should not worry about what we could lose but rather be excited about what we can create and develop for our future.

On top of being more sustainable and peaceful, a vegan society would be healthier, happier, and wealthier! It may sound like a utopia, but no, the science, the data, and the solutions are out there. What would be utopian is to believe we can carry on with the old destructive system.

The Costs of Climate Change

There are a variety of ways that climate change will have an economic impact, some are gradual changes such as increased cooling costs for buildings or rising ocean levels, while others are more dramatic, related to the higher frequency of extreme weather events, such as hurricanes, tornadoes, wildfires, drought or heat waves.

These events which will intensify in strength and frequency are already costing over 200 billion a year in damage for the U.S. alone.[28]

That's only one side of the global warming impact, in a general sense, the economists who study this problem tend to divide the costs up into market and non-market costs. A market cost is a cost to some part of the economy that could be quantified in terms of dollars, while a non-market cost is something that is not easily quantified because there is no market for it. A damaged ecosystem like coral reef is an example of a non-market cost. The damage to reefs has a cost and the cost is probably multifaceted and widespread, but it is not something that can be measured or expressed in dollars.

How much is a healthy Yellow Stone Park worth? The ecosystems and its biomass do not have the technology to prevent, adapt, or quickly repair damages the way humans can. If recurrent wildfires, drought, or extreme weather destroys a nature park, it may not recover for many generations, or at all. A good example is the threat of polar bear extinction.

As the Arctic ice sheet is melting much faster than it used

---

[28] https://feu-us.org/
https://news.nationalgeographic.com/2017/09/climate-change-costs-us-economy-billions-report/

to, polar bears struggle to adapt as they rely on the ice to hunt seals that would otherwise be almost impossible to catch. As a result, polar bears face increasing rates of starvation from not having enough food reserves to survive the warmer season. It is heartbreaking to witness, and we see countless other species impacted by rising temperatures and pollution destroying their habitats.

Nature is ill-equipped to face climate change, and so are poorer nations who will suffer as their governments won't have the resources to face such challenges. Crumbling economies, mass migration, and regional wars might become the norm in a harsher world where natural resources and hospitable land become less available. In the eye of such dire consequences, why not take every possible measure to avert global warming and pollution?

The U.N. believes a global shift toward plant-based food consumption is vital if we are to combat the worst effects of climate change. Globally, animal agriculture is responsible for more greenhouse gases than all the world's transportation systems combined.[29] So, what are we waiting for?

---

[29] http://www.cowspiracy.com/facts

11. ANIMAL GOODS & BY-PRODUCTS

Animal by-products or waste consist of the portion of a slaughtered animal that cannot be sold as meat or used in meat products. Such waste includes bones, tendons, skin, blood, internal organs, and the contents of the gastrointestinal tract. These vary with each type of animal. When an animal is slaughtered, what ends up on the grocery shelves are mainly the muscle parts of the corpse. As you can imagine, breeding over 70 billion land animals plus an estimated 100 billion fish a year creates an unimaginable amount of animal waste non-fit for human consumption. The animal industry had to find ways of monetizing these remaining body parts. Without even realizing it, you probably use at least one item containing inedible animal by-products every day.

Without the income associated with animal by-products, the meat industry could not turn a profit, or the price of meat would skyrocket. This principle goes the other way around too; if they can't sell the meat, the price of the by-products would also skyrocket pushing other industries to find alternatives to replace those raw materials.

This is why, as vegans, it is essential to avoid buying goods that contain animal by-products. Not only do we have a moral responsibility to do so, but it acts as a double edge sword cutting into the profits of the animal exploitation business.

It is almost impossible to avoid all animal by-products as they are virtually everywhere and well hidden in our everyday lives. They are used in the manufacturing of products like industrial lubricant, tires, cosmetics, medicine of all kinds, musical instruments, glue, chewing gum and candies, shampoo and conditioner, brushes, sports equipment, perfume, candles, and detergents to name a few. You would need to live a monk's life on a deserted island to avoid being in touch with these products.

So, what is the best way to start contributing to the decline of animal by-product use? Go with the obvious first. Start by avoiding what your eyes can see like leather in clothing or furniture, down-filled duvets and pillows, wool, cashmere or fur. A wide range of vegan alternatives are easily accessible nowadays.

The next step, which demands a little more awareness is to start reading ingredients in personal care and hygiene products and go for the vegan and cruelty-free option. Aveda, The Body Shop, and Lush are all companies offering a wide selection of vegan beauty and personal care products. Most of them, if plant-based, will usually proudly advertise it on their containers. Veganism is on the rise everywhere around the globe, and these companies are making real efforts to supply animal-friendly customers with high-quality products.

If you do not find vegan versions of your favorite products, please make a request to the store's manager or go online and get in touch with the company's customer service. Money talks. The more demand, the more vegan products will hit the shelves.

As for other products, the best way is to be political about your choices and sometimes go for the lesser of two evils. As I mentioned, it would be almost impossible to avoid animal by-products entirely, but companies are always adjusting to what customers want. If there is demand, requests, and inquiry about vegan products, companies will quickly adapt and provide. It's basic capitalism.

The marketers of those corporations are always scouting customer habits to come out with the most sellable products to get an edge over competitors. They don't care about selling animal by-products or not, as long as they sell a product and turn a profit. It is our responsibility to vote with our purchases and tell those companies what we want. Don't wait for governments or big businesses to act for you; they are both reacting to your actions.

Take the example of fast-food chains like KFC, A&W, Burger King, Carl's Jr, Del Taco, to name a few; they have all recently added vegan plant-based meat substitutes. These changes did not occur out of sudden awareness, but rather because they realized the demand was strong enough. A&W Canada even sold out its Beyond Meat burgers nationwide within weeks of launching it.

Do not underestimate your power as a consumer. A vegan diet in tandem with a reduction of animal by-products consumption is a winning combination to speed up the transition towards a vegan planet.

12. VIVISECTION

"I am not interested to know whether vivisection produces results that are profitable to the human race or doesn't...The pain which it inflicts upon unconsenting animals is the basis of my enmity toward it, and it is to me sufficient justification of the enmity without looking further."

Mark Twain

If vivisection laboratories were practicing on humans instead of animals, we could be medically 25 to 50 years ahead. We could have already found a cure for many diseases, saving millions of adults and children from premature death.

Ninety-five percent of all drugs that are shown to be safe and effective in tests on animals fail in human trials because they don't work or are dangerous. Not only do many medications that work on animals fail in humans, many drugs that could help humans are discarded because they fail in tests on animals.

So, the big question is, why aren't we testing on humans then? The answer is simple: it would be totally immoral. Even to harden criminals or serial killers we could not exercise such cruelty, torment or torture. Instead, we shamefully pick the voiceless, defenseless, innocent ones we can abuse and control. The animals.

Each year, millions of victims, including mice, rats, frogs, dogs, cats, rabbits, hamsters, guinea pigs, monkeys, fish, and birds, are killed in the U.S alone. They die and endure atrocities in laboratories for biology lessons, medical training, chemical, drug, food, and cosmetic testing, and curiosity-driven experimentation.

I was working on a music video promoting veganism recently, and I had to go through hours of vivisection footage to find the right images for the project. Before starting my research, I told myself, "Jeff, you know what you are about to see, you know how bad it will be, so don't get too emotional about it."

Well, it didn't work. The screams, the terror, the agony in their frightened eyes was so disturbing, nothing could have prepared me for it. Every time it hurts, just as much, to be reminded what our society is doing to them: it is soul-crushing. How dare we commit such atrocities?

Imagine for a moment aliens invade the Earth, and you are one of the unlucky to be kidnapped and taken away in their giant spaceship. They take you in their lab to run multiple tests. You do not know where you are, you do not understand their language, nor can they understand you. These enormous 15-foot-tall aliens tower over you, poking and prodding at your skin while you nervously await their next move.

They strip you naked and put you in a cold cage with no comfort whatsoever. You hear other humans screaming in pain, vomiting, and begging for mercy all day and night. After a day or two, one of the aliens walks towards you and opens your cage. You shiver, wet yourself, and beg them to leave you alone.

They grab your arm and force you out, they are much stronger than you; you are defenseless. The alien drags you to a table where he straps your limbs and head, so you can't move or look around. Other aliens come around with strange sharp tools and start touching and measuring your body.

You are petrified. One alien opens your mouth and forces a metal device inside to keep it open. They then insert a tube travelling from your nostrils down to your stomach. You are in immeasurable pain, and though you try to escape, it's in vain. They start pouring an unknown acidic liquid into your mouth. You almost choke to death, but the aliens are indifferent to your suffering.

Your eyes are watering, and your nose is running while you vomit back some of the substance burning your nose and throat. Without care, one of the aliens inserts a catheter in one of your arms. You can't see anything but feel a terrible sting from a needle searching your veins.

One alien unstraps you and forces you back in your cage. You continue vomiting, and trembling in fear, while your stomach burns like fire from the acid. With no water available to you in your cage, you remain completely dehydrated for hours on end.

You are in hell. It is the worst possible situation a sentient being can find themselves in. You are dead to them, and no one cares about you. You don't know what this torture is about or how long it will last. You fret every time an alien passes by your cage, anticipating your turn to be tortured again.

The never-ending screams of other humans, your physical sickness, the confinement of your cage, and your distress makes you lose your mind. You wish you could kill yourself, escape, or wake up from this nightmare but you are stuck in there, and they will keep testing on you until you die. You are completely defeated.

This is what millions of innocent animals imprisoned in labs around the world are going through. These poor animals are tortured to serve humans. We are responsible for our illnesses and way of life, why should any animal suffer for it? There are no excuses, especially as medical technology has advanced considerably, allowing us to draw from computer programs and artificial intelligence for research.[30]

A study led by scientists at Johns Hopkins Bloomberg School of Public Health assert that, "advanced algorithms working from large chemical databases can predict a new chemical's toxicity better than standard animal tests."

It is time to put a stop to this shameful, vile, sadistic horror show and empty those torture chambers. If I didn't convince you with my words today, I invite you to search vivisection on YouTube and decide for yourself. It will shake you to the core.

Please check the labels and buy products that are non-tested on animals. Very often, organic, local, eco-friendly goods

---

[30] https://hub.jhu.edu/2018/07/11/animal-testing-alternative-chemical-database/

from smaller business do not test on animals. Whenever a big brand goes animal cruelty-free, encourage them by selecting those items or boycott if they don't. For us it's such a small effort, for the animals, it means liberation and the end of a nightmare.

13. HUNTING, FISHING & TRAPPING

"Non- violence leads to the highest ethics, which is the goal of all evolution. Until we stop harming all other living beings, we are still savages."

Thomas Alva Edison

Hunting

B eing born in rural Canada, I used to fish, hunt, and even trap. I argued it was necessary to "control" animal populations who could otherwise overpopulate and die of starvation. When I think about it today, it seems completely absurd to kill an animal to save it from dying of overpopulation. What hypocritical reasoning knowing that humans are the only overpopulated animals on earth...

I naively jumped onto that bandwagon firmly believing I was some sort of virtuous ecosystem manager. After all, that's what I was told from an early age. You go to a Canadian outdoor shop, and half the square footage is stocked with hunting or fishing related equipment. Marketing, magazines, local politician support, television programs all portray killing animals as a normal and respectable activity. But when you think about it, killing and loving animals are the complete opposite. Could you love and kill humans as a sport? Could you love and kill dogs with a rifle? Could you love and trap domesticated cats? No, you can't.

When hunters, trappers or fishers are talking about preserving resources or ecosystems, when they picture themselves as "maintaining nature's balance" they are only making sure there is enough prey in the wild to sustain their pastime each year. Like myself at one time, they don't realize modern hunting is a selfish activity resulting in the murder of animals they claim to love and protect.

It is incredible when I look back how blind and disconnected from reality I was. It wasn't about managing natural resources; it was about me. I wasn't hunting, fishing or trapping for any reasons other than my own sadistic pleasure.

I can understand why it is enjoyable to spend time in nature preparing for hunting season. There is a real thrill about tracking your prey's signs of life, finding their territory, and imagining what trophy you could proudly bring home. There is a joy in expressing how skillful, adventurous, and brave you have been in successfully killing the animal.

What we often fail to mention is how the bullet or arrow pierced the defenseless animal's internal organs, causing it to bleed, suffocate, or choke to death in terrible suffering. We also fail to mention many of those victims escape with injuries and die in vain days later. Again, we fail to acknowledge how cowardly we may have killed the animal from the safety of a tree hiding, using technologies that take away any chances the animal has to escape or defend itself.

Killing with Respect

To feel better about their gruesome pastime, hunters or fishers often advocate killing an animal with "respect." They followed the law. They killed within their permit's quota. But is this allocation of catch formulated for the animals, or for the humans to keep killing, year after year without entirely collapsing a species?

In the eyes of hunters or fishers, being respectful also means eating what they kill. Never would they take a life for the sake of taking a life. It's for food. But how can someone possibly take a deer's life for food out of necessity, knowing humans are thriving on a plant-based diet?

Many say eating wild game helps reduce grocery expenses. Reality is, those savings are eradicated by spending on hunting equipment, clothes, permits, gas, accommodations, rifles, or bullets needed to catch wild game.

Whatever the argument, killing sentient beings for a thrill is an action closely linked to psychopathy. If you think the comparison is extreme, how would you call someone shooting dogs and cats in his backyard for entertainment? Social approval, years of publicity, food, and cultural habits have made us blind to the insanity of these activities. They have no place in modern societies.

For some still, those arguments aren't enough, they say it's called the "circle of life". Some say that just like lions, as top predators, we are only expressing our natural hunting instincts.

I could agree with the argument if we were in the 19th

century. Back then, the human population was around one billion, with forests, and oceans mostly intact and teeming with wildlife. I would agree if my survival depended on it. I would agree if, as lions do, we were using fair hunting practices leaving a chance to healthy, strong prey to fight back, escape, reproduce, and pass on their genes. This would be called natural selection. In our time and age, we pride ourselves in killing the bigger, healthier animals while 80% of wildlife populations are in steep decline.

Since most of the wild "game" populations are under sustainable levels, many hunting outfitters have started farming wild species only to release them in the hunting season so that bloodthirsty hunters may have the fun of murdering them. How disturbing and wrong.

Sir **Philip Wollen** former City Bank Vice President and animal right activists describes it best:

"Hunting is an ignoble atrocity; it has no place in a civilized society and to dress it up as sport is an insult to sportsmen's the world over. What sport allow the rules to be determined by only one party? What sport allows only one party to determine the field of play? What sport has the inevitable result of one party dying an agonizing and terrifying death? This is not a sport by any stretch of imagination.

If you really want it to be a sport, there is a solution. Let's get all these brave hunters out into the bush, let them choose their weapons of choice, and with live ammo they can hunt each other. At least there we have the choice; all the parties are there of their own volition. I would like to see people open their eyes to the logic behind banning this disgusting practice. It is not a sport, a past time, the circle of life, or a way of surviving; it is an excuse to a barbaric feast of violence."

If you love nature, spend time in the wild, learn about your favorite animal, track them, and once you spot your prey, and shoot them...with your camera! That's what real animal lovers do.

Fishing

I live in Montreal, Quebec, Canada, a country known for its untouched nature and wilderness. But even here, you now must drive at least four to five hours north to find any lake or river with a healthy population of indigenous fish. Almost all fishing outfitters within this radius and many beyond now rely on fish stocking.

Forget about any wild lakes or rivers easily accessible by roads; they are all mainly overfished. What ever happened to government quotas and fishing permits meant to protect fish stocks? They are simply failing. No natural lakes or rivers can sustain a constant flow of human fishers using technologies like fishing rods, sonars, speed boats, and advanced baiting to fish.

In a human-free environment, very few animals have the skills to feed on fish. With a few exceptions, only otters, some eagles, ducks, and only particular bears can do so. Nature knows how to balance and calibrate the different species together. We clearly don't.

Some will argue that they are respectful since they catch and release to help the fish stock. What if someone was throwing you a sandwich with a hook in it? What if once you have taken a bite, you'd feel a metal hook piercing your jaw, throat, lungs or eyes, while you are pulled underwater?

Once underwater and suffocating, some sea monster violently removes the hook out of your bleeding body, and proudly shows you around to other sea monsters before throwing you back out on to the land unconscious. Would you feel respected? Would you feel the love?

Still, some may argue that since fish are cold-blooded, they don't feel pain. The last time I went fishing, I saw small animals doing everything they could to escape and live. I saw living beings showing unmistakable signs of discomfort and agony. Maybe we don't hear them scream, as they have no vocal cords, but nevertheless who are we to decide if they're suffering, and which levels are acceptable? Who are we to injure or kill a creature that just wanted to live in peace?

If you love lakes or rivers, nothing stops you from leaving your fishing rods behind and enjoying a boat ride. If you are interested in seeing fish, you can always swim with goggles or even scuba dive. It's a fun and insightful way of interacting with the underwater world.

Just this morning, doing my swimming training, I came across a school of Yellow Perch curiously looking at me probably wondering what kind of fish I was! You love fish? Go explore their world, do not violently bring them into yours. Even if they are tiny and much different from us, they are entitled to their lives, just the way we are.

Trapping

Out of hunting and fishing, trapping is undoubtedly the most deceitful and sickening practice. Trapping is mainly done as an economic activity to sell the skin of the animal killed. It once had survival values as we needed the fur to protect ourselves from the cold, but those days are long over.

Once set by the trapper, the traps or snares will indistinctly ambush or kill any animal passing by. Some traps will break bones, or drown their prey, while other types of traps will violently restrain a paw. In the latter case, the animals, on top of acute pain to its limb, may starve to death if the trapper does not come back. In some cases, the trapped animal may get eaten by other animals.

Can you imagine if this was done to you? Can you imagine the distress you would go through? Commonly, some trapped female raccoons, foxes or coyotes will go as far as chewing their own limbs to free themselves to get back to their cubs.

What are we going to do with another species skin anyway? What is so important about it to justify such cruel behaviors? Certainly not save anyone from dying of hypothermia. Instead, the skin will merely end up as fashion garment like on those ugly and shameful Canada Goose winter jackets.

With all the options available to keep warm, how dare we rip the skin off of living beings for a look? How can we not link the dog we love in our home to his cousin coyote murdered for a garment and a trendy label?

Again, it is a total disgrace to trap, and we should see it as nothing short of setting up mines for animals. Fur jackets belong in the past. It is shameful to display such an image of brutality.

Farming fur animals is even worse. Foxes, raccoons, and minks are forced bred and packed in tiny, filthy cages their entire miserable lives only to be electrocuted to death for a garment. Have we gone mad?

It hurts me to walk the streets of Montreal in the wintertime looking at all these fur coats. It is unbelievable that we still have to educate people about such apparent symbols of animal cruelty.

We should also avoid wearing fake fur. Most people can't tell the difference. Wearing fake fur only helps perpetuate the normalization of wearing animal skin.

The World Wildlife Fund (WWF) for Nature's Living Planet report released in 2018, describes a worldwide catastrophic decline in animal populations. Well over half the world's population of vertebrates, from fish to birds to mammals, have been wiped out in the past four decades. Between 1970 and 2014, there was a 60 percent decline, among 16,700 wildlife populations around the world according to the report.[31]

Humans now account for about 36 percent of the biomass of all mammals, livestock for 60 percent, and wild mammals for only four percent. Shouldn't we leave the four percent alone and do everything in our power to protect them?

---

[31] https://www.nationalgeographic.com/animals/2018/11/animal-decline-living-planet-report-conservation-news/

14. CULTURAL HERITAGE

"People often say that humans have always eaten animals, as if this is some justification for continuing the practice. According to this logic, we should not try to prevent people from murdering other people, since this has also been done since the earliest of times."

Isaac Bashevis Singer

I was recently having a conversation over the killing of whales in the Faroe Islands. It was argued this tradition should be respected and that nothing was wrong with killing whales for food, and that only in the eyes of vegan extremists was such hunting seen as immoral.

Each year in this self-governing archipelago, part of the Kingdom of Denmark, thousands of pilot whales, beaked whales and dolphins are chased into the bay by boats, where they are slaughtered.

Metal hooks are driven into the stranded mammals' blowholes before their spines are cut. The animals slowly bleed to death. Whole families are murdered, and some whales swim around in their family members' blood for hours. It is a gruesome scene. There is so much blood in the water that the bay turns red. Whales and dolphins are highly intelligent creatures, and as mammals, they feel pain just as much as we do.

Locals defend the practice as being part of their culture for hundreds of years. They also claim whale meat is an essential source of food even though whale meat is eaten only a couple of times a month, not more, because of the high mercury content that accumulates in the animal from feeding on other fish.

So, the question is, should we in 2019, with an overpopulated earth, and declining ocean ecosystems carry on with such violent traditions with a plentiful supply of plant-based food? Should the whales suffer the cost of an ever-expanding human population and their choice of settlement? Food may be scarce on the Faroe Islands, but when there are numerous alternatives to whale meat, why should another species suffer the consequences?

It is also interesting to point out the words "respect," and "choice" are often used by meat-eaters in their arguments to go about their business. If it is so important to them, then what about respecting the whales and their decision to live? It seems the animals, regarding their own life, do not have that choice.

We live in an ever-changing world where cultures evolve. Be they cruel or just plain odd by today's standards, many cultural practices of the past would be incomprehensible or unacceptable today.

Cultural heritage or holy book writings are no excuse to carry on with obsolete practices. Whale hunting, corridas, farm factories, horse carriage rides, donkey transportation, and animal circus' will eventually be seen for what they are: senseless acts of violence and slavery.

As an intelligent species, I invite you to think critically and question yourself: are these traditions, centuries-old or not, aligned with a modern society's values? Aligned with my own values? Do I partake in traditions that cause needless suffering?

15. PETS & PET FOOD

"If you love someone, set them free. If they come back, they're yours; if they don't, they never were"

Richard Bach

Pets

Have you ever watched the classic Tchaikovsky production Swan Lake? It tells the story of Odette, a princess turned into a swan by an evil sorcerer's curse. The sorcerer was so in love with the princess he kept her captive in a golden suspended prison to force her to fall in love with him. The moral of this beautiful piece is you do not jail whom you love.

Animals are no different than Odette. When you walk into a pet shop, you meet many animal "lovers" looking to buy different exotic species like fish, birds, or reptiles. Those customers may have good intentions and genuinely believe they love animals, but are they behaving like the sorcerer by imprisoning whom they "love"?

From an early age, society has taught us that keeping a sentient being in a cage is acceptable, but let's think about this for a moment.

Any animal in a pet shop has been forced bred or captured from their natural environment for a profit, not out of love. Just like industrial farming, the tragedies happening behind the scene are well concealed. A pet shop is not as cute, or entertaining as it may look, it is indeed, an animal slaves' market. Am I going too far?

What about the history of these animals? What about their mothers and fathers, what about the decimation of the wild population and poaching due to this commerce? What about the stress imposed on these animals? Their living conditions? Their treatment? How many of them died in the process?

Take the example of parrots. Because of their popularity, we capture them from the jungle, cut the feathers from their wings, throw them in cages and sell them to humans for personal entertainment. The cages are usually just big enough for the bird to spread what remains of their wingspan.

If you compare to human size, imagine being jailed for the rest of your life in a cell about 10x10 feet. The bird, who was born to fly in flocks for miles a day, is now confined to stand on a wooden pole, day in day out, alone. For a highly sociable animal, what a sad state of living, and what an unjust jail sentence from an "animal lover".

The parrot has no freedom, eats the same food every day. It has no social interaction with other birds, no courting, no sexuality, no family. As a species that's meant to freely roam the skies, it is subjected to complete boredom and confinement. Is this love?

If you have to keep an animal in a tank, a cage, a vivarium or any other type of confinement, it means the animal should be free.

If you truly love a certain species, protect their environment, buy yourself the equipment you need to visit them in the wild. Take pictures or videos to share with your friends. Fish belong to oceans, birds to the sky, and reptiles to the deserts. They do not belong to a prison in a human living room.

As for dogs and cats and other domesticated animals, a pet shop should be the last place you go to find a new family member. Animal shelters are crowded with loving cats and dogs deserving a new home. You could be their last chance at finding a family.

Each year, approximately 1.5 million shelter animals are euthanized via gas chambers (670,000 dogs and 860,000 cats) in the U.S alone.[32] Getting a cat or a dog is a life-long commitment, how can we get rid of 125,000 of those loyal companions every month as if they were disposable things?

There are exceptions where it is necessary to send an animal to a shelter, but they are a fraction of those numbers. Most of these victims are bought without much forethought into the responsibility and time an animal family member requires.

Moving out, boyfriend's allergy, behavioral issues, lack of time are no excuses to shatter your loyal animal's heart and unfeelingly send them to their death. Pets are not

---

[32] https://www.aspca.org/animal-homelessness/shelter-intake-and-surrender/pet-statistics

expendable goods. You should only adopt a domestic animal if you have comprehensively accepted the lifelong responsibility that comes with it.

Pet food

I have two adorable, playful Jack Russell Parson's, Solo and Suki. I got the first one, from an individual who had a litter of pups and the second one, is a rescue from a family who didn't want to deal with a dog anymore. I have had them for over eight years now.

In the beginning, I was mainly feeding them regular fish-based dry food. But as a vegan, I was always uncomfortable with killing animals weekly to keep mine alive. It was a paradox, but I thought I didn't have much choice. I believed dogs could not live on a vegan diet.

That was before I met a friend who told me dogs were omnivores who can thrive on plant-based food. I did my research and indeed found lots of information and examples that confirmed it.

I gave it a try, and it is now almost four years since my dogs had their last piece of animal flesh and they are both healthy and in great shape. Solo and Suki are my best training partners jogging half marathons with me on a regular basis.

I have since learned that If you have been feeding your companion animal regular commercial dry food, you may be jeopardizing their health. Supermarket pet foods are often made up of farmed animals deemed unfit for human consumption by the U.S. Department of Agriculture. These animals usually fall into one of these categories: dead before slaughterhouse, dying, diseased, or disabled.[33]

Many of these animals have died of infections and other diseases. If you are concerned about your pet's health and the cruelty of the meat industry, you may want to stop buying meat-based commercial pet food.

Image you bring home a dead raccoon you found on the highway. Its bloated, smelly body indicates that it likely died a couple of days ago. Placing the decaying body in a pot, you boil it for a couple of hours to kill any bacteria, and parasites. After draining the water, you grind up the boiled corpse with chemical products that divide protein from fat. You turn the protein into a flour you can use in many recipes and use the fat as a spread for your morning toast. This is basically what we are serving our pets. Though the process has rendered the raccoon comestible, is it really what you want to feed your beloved animal companions?

I'm not saying dogs are not fine eating meat, they are, I'm saying the quality of the meat and the list of ingredients in most commercial pet food is highly questionable. For the purists who think it is very unnatural to serve a plant-based meal to a dog, let me remind you that there is nothing natural about dry food either.

I have discovered that more and more vegans feed healthful, meatless diets to their companion animals. One remarkable example is that of Bramble, a 27-year-old border collie whose vegan diet of rice, lentils, and organic vegetables earned her consideration by the Guinness Book of World

[33]https://www.petmd.com/dog/nutrition/evr_pet_food_for_your_pets_sake

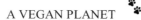

Records as the world's oldest living dog in 2002.[34]

Cats are often more finicky than dogs, and their nutritional requirements are more complicated. Though my personal experience with cats is limited, I can suggest the book "Vegetarian Cats & Dogs" by James Peden. Peden also developed a product called, "Vegepet™" which are supplements to add to your furry friend's vegan meals. They are nutritionally balanced and come in special formulas for kittens, puppies, and lactating cats and dogs. Always consult with your veterinarian prior to changing your pet's food.

---

[34] https://www.bordercolliefanclub.com/bramble-the-vegan-dog-lives-to-189-years/

16. PEACE OF MIND & SPIRITUALITY

"For as long as men massacre animals, they will kill each other. Indeed, he who sows the seed of murder and pain cannot reap joy and love."

Pythagoras

Humans have a godlike power over all animals and their habitats. We are feared by all, and no other creature on this Earth can possibly compete with us. Our survival has long been secured.

Isn't it time we change our attitudes and become a gentle force protecting and supporting our animal relatives? Wouldn't we all feel better about ourselves knowing we have evolved from destructing, to helping who we share this planet with? Haven't we taken enough already from animals?

In previous chapters, we have discussed the differences between living a vegan and non-vegan way of life. We have seen how our choices can make the difference between compassion or cruelty, health or sickness, protecting or destroying ecosystems, and economic gains or losses.

But what about the intangible impacts of a non-vegan life such as our mental wellbeing, and spirituality? What could we gain in terms of justice, peace of mind, and happiness?

If we could decide, what kind of world would we choose to live in?

If I asked a crowd of a thousand people "who loves animals?" the vast majority would raise their hands. Then, if I asked, "who is against animal cruelty?" the vast majority would raise their hands. Finally, if I asked, "who condemns non-necessary violence or abuse to animals or humans?" Again, the vast majority would raise their hands.

We all have a strong sense of justice and compassion within us. It explains why we can't bear watching videos of animal or human cruelty. A child can tell the fundamental difference between right or wrong. We are born with this ability.

There are countless videos online where you see children pleading to save the life of their animal friends who are about to be slaughtered. It is instinctual not to hurt a sentient being who does not pose a threat or otherwise exhibit signs of danger.

But as we age, our mind, like a sponge, absorbs all kinds of information burying our innate compassion and making us behave in ways that contradict our very nature. We learn over time to accept animal violence as being normal. Even if deep inside we know our actions are less than righteous, we take comfort in social acceptance to turn a blind eye.

Unconsciously, could such unnatural behavior lead to anxiety? Could sponsoring violence with our daily consumption lead to a subtle, yet ever-present sense of guilt? Could refusing to acknowledge the unnecessary cruelty of our way of life be causing some mental distress?

The harrowing psychological toll of slaughterhouse workers has been well documented. If a pig came and nuzzled you like a puppy, would you be able to stab it to death just moments later? This is one of the scenarios faced by slaughterhouse workers daily. They kill animals that are no different to those we welcome into our homes as family members. Hundreds, sometimes thousands of them a day.

The psychological toll this takes on a person cannot be underestimated. Slaughterhouse work has been linked to a variety of disorders, including PTSD (post-traumatic stress disorder). Slaughterhouse work has also been connected to an increase in crime rates, including higher incidents of domestic abuse, as well as alcohol and drug abuse.[35]

As consumers buying a packaged product at the end of the food chain, we can avoid the dirty job. We don't have to kill the pig we eat in our sandwiches. But, with increased awareness of what the animals are going through, with the endless stream of animal cruelty videos on our social media and news feed, how can we not feel, to at least some degree, responsible or guilty for the victims?

How can we not make the connection between our money and the slaughterhouse worker's knife? And when we do connect, when we become aware even for just a moment, one cannot help but feel embarrassed and sad for what animals are made to endure. We realize we should change but somehow, we don't follow through, we go back to our routine of hollow justification and try to forget.

This emotional discomfort is like a little rock in a shoe,

---

[35] https://www.ncbi.nlm.nih.gov/pmc/articles/PMC4841092/

constantly aggravating you. What price are we paying on a psychological level for our meat addiction?

If we believe in social justice and compassion for all, how can we possibly eat violence three times a day? If we are against slavery, racism, violence against women, child abuse, or any other great social cause, how can we stand so blind and selfish in the face of this animal holocaust?

If you believe in karma, humans are indebting themselves for generations to come. In this life or another, I have the feeling we'll have to face the consequences of our actions.

We are spiritual beings seeking love and happiness; what are we doing walking this path of destruction? We are one with this planet; ultimately, we are destroying ourselves.

I understand it is impossible to resolve all world issues overnight. We may feel powerless regarding regional wars in Africa, labor camps in North Korea, or widespread poverty around the world, but there is something we can easily act upon right away; our diet. Three times a day we can act for our future. Three times a day we can save animal lives, precious drinking water, and forests. Believe me, the feeling of being part of the solution by far, outweighs any small inconvenience of adjusting your food habits.

You can lead by example to the people around you who will then in time, follow your lead. Even though the old system may continue for a while, you can sleep at night knowing you are no longer part of it. What matters is not necessarily winning but trying our best.

Wouldn't it feel great to know humanity is shifting with a

sense of urgency towards reshaping our future and our destiny for the better? It all starts with one individual action, one little adjustment in our daily routine to create a global shift towards an exciting future. Rest assured: it is not too late. We have time, we have the tools, and the technology to turn things around and make this world a better one.

17. ACTIVISM

"The world will not be destroyed by those who do evil, but by those who watch them without doing anything."

Albert Einstein

Have you ever watched a video on YouTube or in the news where someone is in obvious danger and bystanders do nothing? Did you feel frustrated they didn't help? Do you think you would have acted differently?

Have you ever wondered why the German population allowed Nazi-led death camps to exist? Would you have raised your voice against black slavery if you were living in the 19th century?

Well, that feeling, or questioning is what activism is all about. It is about taking action to stop exploitation and injustice. Activism is not selling a cult, products, or a trend, it is about raising awareness to ongoing issues that demand change. It is about having the courage to stand up for what you believe is right.

Vegan activism takes many forms. It could be as simple as having conversations with family, friends, or colleagues. It could take the form of social media posts. It could be participating in organized street protests, storming a fur shop, or exposing industrial farms or slaughterhouses.

Some will be touched by reading books, while others will connect with videos and imagery. Some may be more influenced by extraordinary actions that catch the mainstream media's attention. All these actions are equally valuable to defend a cause when non-violent.

I'm firmly against aggressive street demonstrations, destroying random shops, fighting police officers or anything of the sort. I prefer relying on people's heart and common sense when passing a message.

That being said, in the pursuit of a greater good, I fully agree with the philosophy behind one having a moral responsibility to disobey unjust laws. Civil disobedience is sometimes warranted. Being a good citizen is not always the same thing as being a good person.

By refusing to give up her seat to a white person on a Montgomery, Alabama city bus in 1955, black seamstress Rosa Parks helped initiate the civil rights movement in the United States.

The great Mohandas Gandhi's defiance of British colonial laws over the empire's salt monopoly, beginning in March 1930, sparked a wave of civil disobedience leading to India's independence from the British Empire.

There are clear parallels with animal liberation activists today. We must peacefully but firmly demonstrate veganism is a revolution that cannot be stopped before the day the last cage is empty, slaughterhouses are out of business, and meat consumption is a thing of the past.

New movement leaders are often criticized or labeled as

extremists or anarchists. It is a strategy by the establishment to invalidate the legitimacy or foundation behind the activist's actions or goals. Do not listen or fall for the way some media or lobbyists describe vegans. Vegans are not "extremist", it is never extreme to ask for compassion and the end of useless violence.

It is not extreme to break in hidden industrial complexes to show the world the atrocious conditions animals are living in. What is extreme is having billions of victims as lovely and smart as the pets we love imprisoned and tortured for a profit. That is extreme. To the contrary, the brave activists taking risks to defend the voiceless are true leaders deserving of recognition.

It is impossible to name all activists out there, but if you would like to learn more about veganism and get inspired, here is a list of some amazing and outstanding people I follow:

Sir Philip Wollen

Former Vice-President of Citibank, Wollen conducts intervention programs to rescue abused animals and funds outreach programs that promote animal welfare. He is a gifted writer and public speaker. You can read one of his inspiring speeches featured at the end of this book.

Ed Winters

He is a vegan educator, public speaker, and content creator based in London, England. Winters is the co-founder and co-director of Surge, an animal rights organization determined to create a world where compassion towards all non-human animals is the norm. Ed is known for his peaceful communication approach with the public on sensitive topics. Visit earthlinged.org to learn more about him and his work.

James Aspey

In January 2014, this animal welfare activist from Australia pledged not to speak for 365 days, hoping that, in his voice lessness, he could draw attention to the plight of the millions of animals on the planet raised for human consumption. He has since been very outspoken and active on the scene. You can find Aspey on Instagram @jamesaspey.

Gary Yourofsky

An American animal rights activist and lecturer pioneer. Yourofsky has given speeches to thousands of college students. He has had a significant influence on contemporary veganism. He spent 77 days in a Canadian maximum-security prison in 1999, after raiding a fur farm in Canada and releasing 1,542 minks in 1997 that were due to be skinned for fashion. Visit https://www.adaptt.org/ to read more.

Erin Janus

Janus has produced many educational and impactful videos on veganism. One of them called, "Dairy is Scary" has reached millions of views and made it to 60 billboards across California. This articulate and short video captures the horrors of the dairy industry for both animals and humans. Follow her Facebook page to learn more about her work by searching Erin Janus.

Joey Carbstrong

Carbstrong is an activist who is not afraid to tell things as they are. He has been invited on several TV and radio shows to defend his comments associating animal farming with rape, murder, and slave ownership. He has faced off with TV host Piers Morgan who labeled vegans "terrorists". For more information visit joeycarbstrong.com.

Leah Doellinger

Known for her brave activism, Doellinger has saved countless animals from factory farms and has faced arrests and other legal consequences in the name of animal liberty. Doellinger has the courage that very few have by breaking into industrial farms to create content that exposes the horrific conditions animals live in. You can follow Doellinger on Instagram @leahdoellinger.

George Martin

He is the founder of Carnism Debunked and organizer for Anonymous for the Voiceless. Instead of using images or videos, Martin mainly uses his words to create thoughtful content bringing the readers to reflect on some of their beliefs and food habits.

Follow him on Instagram @george_martin_ar or visit his website www.carnismdebunked.com which offers some of the best answers to debunk carnism.

Rich Roll

Last but not least, Roll is a 50-year old accomplished vegan ultra-endurance athlete and former entertainment attorney turned full-time wellness & plant-based nutrition advocate. Popular public speaker, his podcast inspires millions of people worldwide. You will be amazed by his incredible journey. Visit richroll.com to learn more.

PETA

I would like to put a word in acknowledging The People for the Ethical Treatment of Animals (PETA). For almost 40 years, this amazing non-profit organization has relentlessly worked towards the promotion of a vegan lifestyle and animal liberation.

I would also like to address past accusations claiming PETA has staged false content of animal cruelty. Nowadays, with the thousands of existing videos exposing animal abuse from science labs to industrial farms, it is clear such accusations were nonsense and only aimed at discrediting PETA. I highly recommend visiting their website at www.peta.org where you can find useful information about veganism.

Activists are playing a pivotal role in uncovering, documenting, and publicly sharing the hidden misery animals are going through. It is their often-anonymous work that is giving us the proof through images and videos we need in our argument for a plant-based world.

To be on site and witness the gruesome conditions of these animals with your own eyes is profoundly shocking. Even more disturbing for activists, is coming face to face with the darker side of humanity and trying to remain hopeful. It is trying to understand why otherwise kind and caring people continue to participate in needless violence against animals.

I want to take the opportunity to thank every single one of them for making this world a better one. You are the early, unsung heroes of the greatest revolution of our history.

Animals are voiceless, and defenseless. They have no government representing them, no lawyers, or associations. If we don't voice our concerns for them, who will? I used to say; "I'm vegan but I respect your choice of eating meat," until the day I realized we were forgetting someone here. As I mentioned in the chapter about cultural heritage, if freedom of choice is so important, then what about the animal's choice to live and not suffer?

In fact, by accepting someone else's choice to hurt animals, I was protecting myself from the judgment of my peers. By putting my social status and opinions of others first, I was turning a blind eye on something I knew was wrong. I was the bystander who did nothing to help. I didn't want to be judged, mocked at, or uninvited to my friend's next BBQ. I didn't want to be portraited as an "extremist" for speaking the truth.

No one would respect someone's choice to abuse kids, to act violently towards women, or mistreat a dog or cat. So how can we accept madness of such magnitude when it comes to animals forced-bred into hellish factory farms?

If a child was caught killing or torturing an animal for the pleasure of it, it's most likely the parents would seek advice from a psychologist or thoroughly question their kid as such behavior would be very disturbing. So how can we, as adults, accept to kill and torture for the taste of bacon or a fashion garment? Bacon is nothing but a few seconds of pleasure; it is certainly not needed in any healthy diet, and yet we are ok with murdering for it.

Animal exploitation is barbaric just like the exploitation of any human being. The only difference is animal exploitation is coated with marketing and social approval. Pain and suffering are not exclusive to humans. Murder is murder, rape is rape and a victim is a victim. We have a moral duty to raise our voices and speak the truth. We can no longer remain complicit in accepting the unacceptable.

When family, friends, and co-workers, hear your arguments, when they see your determination, they may dismiss, ridicule, or even reject you at first. But believe me, you are planting seeds in their mind that only grow with time.

Nobody wants to be cruel to animals. Nobody wants to destroy the planet. Nobody wants to get sick. Most people are simply unwilling to give up their bad habits, but this is where you can help them.

In 2019, a vegan lifestyle is accessible, easy, and delicious. Anyone can do it. By firmly voicing your concerns, you are helping other people around you make a positive change in their lives. Everyone will win the sooner this planet turns vegan. Do not be afraid, be brave, and speak the truth from your heart.

18.

VEGAN ATHLETES & CELEBRITIES

"I've found that a person does not need protein from meat to be a successful athlete. My best year of track competition was the first year I ate a vegan diet."

Carl Lewis

As the virtues of a plant-based diet are becoming more and more prevalent each year, some high-level athletes, and celebrities have started taking notes. Almost every week we hear of new singers, actors, businesspeople, politicians or influencers becoming vegan. Here is my 2019, top 10 list of the most influential vegan athletes and celebrities. Let's learn a little more about them and the reason behind their life-changing choices.

Tom Brady

The New England Patriots quarterback Tom Brady and his wife, supermodel Gisele Bündchen, enjoy a vegan diet. American football is a sport of hard work and brute strength. How remarkable the football player many sports analysts consider to be the greatest quarterback of all time thrives on a vegan diet. One would think football players would be the most conservative about meat-eating, but it seems mentalities are evolving. Here is a quote from an article on the subject from CNBC dated Jan 2018. Coming from the American Football world, it's worth a read.[36]

"NFL players' surprising new performance hack; going vegan!

When you think of what NFL players eat, you might imagine hulking athletes tearing into juicy steaks and scarfing fattening food. Perhaps it's not so far from the truth: ESPN recently reported it takes nearly 600 pounds of beef to feed the Buffalo Bills for a week, and that's not even counting chicken (700 pounds) and fish. And who can forget that hot dog-and-Cheetos dinner Jacksonville Jaguars' Jalen Ramsey once tweeted?

However, for an increasing number of players, that's changing. With quarterback Tom Brady headed to his eighth Super Bowl with the New England Patriots on Sunday, others in the league have taken notice of his healthy habits. As the Boston Globe points out: "It's a movement being led by Tom Brady, who dominated the league in his late 30s and is still going strong at 40, thanks to his vegetable-based diet and flexibility training over muscle mass."

And now, there's a new performance hack taking hold in the NFL; going vegan. Brady himself teamed up with vegan meal delivery service Purple

---

[36] https://www.cnbc.com/2018/09/07/nfl-players-are-going-vegan.html

Carrot to create a meatless, dairy-free TB12 performance meal plan in 2016. And this season, the Tennessee Titans had a reported 11 team members go vegan ("with varying levels of commitment," according to ESPN). The team made it all the way to the playoffs for the first time in a decade, reports SI.com."

If the American Football world can open their mind to veganism, anyone can!

Venus Williams

When Venus Williams was diagnosed with Sjogren's syndrome in 2011, her tennis career almost came to a grinding halt. After a rough season of injuries and match withdrawals, she announced that she was suffering from the fairly common autoimmune disease that causes dry eye and dry mouth, as well as crushing joint pain and fatigue.

The condition severely hindered her athletic performance, ultimately leaving her no choice but to withdraw from the 2011 U.S. Open in the second round. But after taking time off, Williams was able to step back onto the court with newfound strength, thanks to proper treatment, and, you guessed it: a drastic diet change. She began following a raw vegan diet.

Lewis Hamilton

Formula One World Champion, Lewis Hamilton, has said he is healthier and happier than ever before on a vegan diet. Last year he blasted the meat industry for animal torture on Instagram, saying:

"Every bit of meat, chicken, or fish you eat, every bit of leather or fur you wear, has come from an animal that has been tortured, pulled away from their families and brutally killed. We all have choices to make, and if you are ok with it, then that's you, but I choose to love, to be conscious of what I'm supporting and I refuse to support the companies that buy from those companies killing and torturing animals."

"Iron" Mike Tyson

Yes, you read that right. The former undisputed world heavyweight champion, who was the youngest person ever to win the title at just 20 years old, has been vegan for many years.

When Tyson was questioned as to whether he could have followed a plant-based diet during his fighting days, he admitted he was unsure, but pointed out that "the greatest gladiators, the greatest ones in Roman times, they were all vegan. That's fighting to the death!"

Xavier Desharnais

I want to conclude the vegan athlete section by talking about my friend Xavier Desharnais, a Canadian long-distance open water swimming champion. Believing in the plant-based diet nutrient benefits and animal welfare, Desharnais, went against his coach's advice and most of his entourage by turning vegan in 2012.

Following his new food habit, he went on to finish second at the Lac Memphremagog World Cup, a 34km distance, in

2012 and 2013. In 2014 and 2015, he won first place at the international 32km Lac St-Jean race. He finished the same race in 2018, only 0.7 seconds behind the winner. In 2015, Xavier was ranked top three worldwide for men's endurance swimming. He has competed in races all over the world including the Santa Fe-Coronda in Argentina, a 57km long competition.

Swimming the Ironman distance of 3.8km is already hard enough: I can only imagine how much endurance is needed to swim such distances. Desharnais is another vegan athlete showing us how much we can thrive on a plant-based diet.

Ariana Grande

Ariana has been vegan since 2013 after realizing she loved animals too much to hurt them. "I love animals more than I love most people, not kidding," said the talented pop singer. Since she announced her choice to follow a vegan diet, she's been a prominent animal rights activist.

Joaquin Phoenix

This Oscar-nominated actor was offered several big commercial breaks in adverts for meat and milk products when he started his career but turned them down. The talented actor by-passed the cheesy commercial world entirely. Now, he's a world-famous movie star, still a vegan, and an ambassador for animal cruelty prevention charity, PETA.

Bryan Adams

Canadian-born rock star Bryan Adams has two very different sides to his life; making stadium anthems and campaigning for Greenpeace and PETA. "I've made a conscious decision not to be part of the cycle of killing animals because I couldn't see the point of crusading for Greenpeace and then eating a fish. Seriously, if you are going to talk the talk, you need to walk the walk," he said.

Bill Clinton

Former U.S. President Bill Clinton was named PETA's Person of 2010 after he began promoting the benefits of vegan eating. He changed his habits for health reasons, and thanks to the plant-based diet, he shed a whopping 24lbs.

Brad Pitt

Although it's not precisely known when Brad Pitt turned vegan, he has been an animal activist for a very long time. He has been actively supporting social causes and has also been working on many environmental issues for years. Amongst the list of most influential people in the world, his approach towards organic and vegan living has inspired many of his fans and co-stars.

James Cameron

Cameron has followed a vegan diet himself since 2011 and hopes that his new feature-length film "the game changer", will help show how beneficial a vegan diet can be from both a personal and global perspective. The film features vegan Olympic athletes, bodybuilders, F1 world champion Lewis

Hamilton and NFL's Tennessee Titans football team.

He explained that one of his main intentions with The Game Changers is to promote veganism to men by debunking the common misconception that a vegan diet is always insufficient in protein. The film does this by highlighting the myriad plant-based proteins available and interviewing a whole host of famously "bulky" vegans, such as Arnold Schwarzenegger.

In a recent interview, the Ontario-born director said, "More than that, I think that if we don't make a major shift as a civilization, and I mean that globally, towards plant-based eating, we're just not going to make it. We can't keep consuming Earth like we've got four more of them standing behind it."

As I'm writing this book, the film is expected to be released at some point in 2019. Being passionate about health and sport myself, I cannot wait to watch it. Even if there are many excellent vegan documentaries out there it's the first one, to my knowledge, to have such a legendary producer behind it. Indeed, after Titanic and Avatar's success, one can hope the Game Changer will become a game changer for veganism!

19.   CONCLUSION

"The greatness of a nation and its moral progress can be judged by the way in which its animals are treated. I hold that the more helpless a creature, the more entitled it is to protection by man from the cruelty of man."

Gandhi

I wrote the last chapters of the book, Frequently Asked Questions, Nutrients, Grocery List and One-Week Meal Plan as reference sections or memorandum you can come back to as often as needed. But, before you jump into the recipes or learn about the practical answers of the frequently asked questions chapter, in conclusion of this book, I would like to leave you with one of my favorite speeches.

It is written by vegan activist and former Citibank Vice President, Sir Philip Wollen. His eloquence, righteousness, and sense of justice is profoundly touching. His inspiring speech given at St. James Ethics and the Wheeler Centre debate, has driven me to further my involvement for the animal cause.

I strongly recommend you watching his speech on Youtube[37] his delivery is very empowering.

---

[37] https://www.youtube.com/watch?v=uQCe4qEexjc&t=146s

Congratulations! Reading this page means you have invested time and effort into learning more about veganism and its many great possibilities. I have finally put years of observations and reflection into words, and I thank you from the bottom of my heart for allowing me to share it with you.

My main motivation for writing this book was to raise awareness, and I hope I succeeded in inspiring you to embark upon a plant-based way of life.

It is now your turn to take the lead and make a difference in the world.

GO VEGAN and thrive my friend!

With love and gratitude,

Jeff &

20. PHILIP WOLLEN'S WORDS

King Lear, late at night on the cliffs asks the blind Earl of Gloucester:

"How do you see the world?"

And the blind man Gloucester replies, "I see it feelingly."

Shouldn't we all?

Animals must be off the menu because tonight they are screaming in terror in the slaughterhouses, in crates, and in cages; vile ignoble gulags of despair.

I heard the screams of my dying father as his body was ravaged by the cancer that killed him. And I realized I had heard these screams before.

In the slaughterhouse, eyes stabbed out, and tendons slashed, on the cattle ships to the Middle East and the dying mother whale as a Japanese harpoon explodes in her brain as she calls out to her calf.

Their cries were the cries of my father.

I discovered when we suffer; we suffer as equals.

And in their capacity to suffer, a dog is a pig, is a bear, is a boy.

Meat is the new asbestos, more murderous than tobacco.

CO_2, Methane, and Nitrous Oxide from the livestock industry are killing our oceans with acidic, hypoxic dead zones.

Ninety percent of small fish are ground into pellets to feed livestock.

Vegetarian cows are now the world's largest ocean predator.

The oceans are dying in our time. By 2048 all our fisheries will be dead. The lungs and the arteries of the Earth.

Billions of bouncy little chicks are ground up alive simply because they are male.

Only 100 billion people have ever lived. 7 billion alive today. And yet we torture and kill two billion animals every week.

Ten thousand entire species are wiped out every year because of the actions of one species.

We are now facing the sixth mass extinction in cosmological history.

If any other organism did this, a biologist would call it a virus.

It is a crime against humanity of unimaginable proportions.

The world has changed.

Ten years ago, Twitter was a bird sound, www was a stuck keyboard, Cloud was in the sky, 4 g was a parking place, Google was a baby burp, Skype was a typo, and Al Qaida was my plumber.

Victor Hugo said, "there is nothing more powerful than an idea whose time has come."

Animal rights is now the greatest social justice issue since the abolition of slavery.

There are over 600 million vegetarians in the world.

That is bigger than the US, England, France, Germany, Spain, Italy, Canada, Australia combined! If we were one nation, we would be bigger than the 27 countries in the European Union!

Despite this massive footprint, we are still drowned out by the raucous huntin', shootin', killin' cartels who believe that violence is the answer when it shouldn't even be a question.

Meat is a killing industry, animals, us and our economies.

Medicare has already bankrupted the United States. They will need eight trillion invested in Treasury bills just to pay the interest. They have precisely zero!

They could shut every school, army, navy, air force, and homeland security, Marines, the CIA and FBI they still won't be able to pay for it.

Cornell and Harvard say that the optimum amount of meat for a healthy diet is precisely ZERO.

Water is the new oil. Nations will soon be going to war for it.

Underground aquifers that took millions of years to fill are running dry.

It takes 15,000 liters of water to produce one kilo of beef.

One billion people today are hungry. Twenty million people will die from malnutrition. Cutting meat by only 10% will feed 100 million people. Eliminating meat will end starvation forever.

If everyone ate a Western diet, we would need two Planet Earths to feed them. We only have one. And she is dying.

Greenhouse gas from livestock is 50% more than transport, planes, trains, trucks, cars, and ships.

Poor countries sell their grain to the West while their own children starve in their arms. And we feed it to livestock. So we can eat a steak? Am I the only one who sees this as a crime? Every morsel of meat we eat is slapping the tear-stained face of a starving child. When I look into her eyes, should I be silent?

The Earth can produce enough for everyone's need. But not enough for everyone's greed.

We are facing the perfect storm.

If any nation had developed weapons that could wreak such havoc on the planet, we would launch a pre-emptive military strike and bomb it into the Bronze Age.

But it is not a rogue state. It is an industry.

The good news is we don't have to bomb it. We can just

stop buying it.

George Bush was wrong. The Axis of Evil doesn't run through Iraq, Iran or North Korea. It runs through our dining tables. Weapons of Mass Destruction are our knives and forks.

Our proposition is the Swiss Army Knife of the future. It solves our environmental, water, health problems and ends cruelty forever.

The Stone Age didn't end because we ran out of stones. This cruel industry will end because we run out of excuses.

Meat is like 1 and 2 cent coins. It costs more to make than it is worth.

And farmers are the ones with the most to gain. Farming won't end. It would boom. Only the product line would change. Farmers would make so much money they wouldn't even bother counting it.

Governments will love us. New industries would emerge and flourish. Health insurance premiums would plummet. Hospital waiting lists would disappear.

Hell "We'd be so healthy; we'd have to shoot someone just to start a cemetery!"

Animals are not just other species. They are other nations. And we murder them at our peril.

The peace map is drawn on a menu. Peace is not just the absence of war. It is the presence of justice.

Justice must be blind to race, color, religion, or species. If she is not blind, she will be a weapon of terror. And there is unimaginable terror in those ghastly Guantanamos we call factory farms or slaughterhouses.

If slaughterhouses had glass walls, we wouldn't need this debate.

I believe another world is possible.

On a quiet night, I can hear her breathing.

Let's get the animals off the menu and out of these torture chambers.

---

21. FREQUENTLY ASKED QUESTIONS

As you take your first steps towards veganism and tell your family and social circle about your new habits, you are very likely to induce some debates and questioning. It is normal, as we eat three times a day, everyone seems compelled by diet discussions. Do not worry, I understand we have covered many subjects with a lot of data throughout this book, it's a considerable amount of information to remember. So, to give you the best possible start and the tools to shine at your next family dinner, I wrote the frequently asked questions section for you to use as a reference. I wrote simple, straightforward answers to the most common questions or misconceptions you may come across.

Where do you get your protein?

I get my protein from the same place animals with the biggest muscles such as bulls, elephants, horses or gorillas do; from plants. Nuts, legumes, beans, seeds, tofu all have similar or more protein per gram than meat.

What do you eat as a vegan?

Fruits, vegetables, nuts, legumes, grains, seeds, bread, pasta, tofu, tempeh are the basis on which to build recipes. Most of my favorite meat dishes can easily be made vegan.

For example; meatball spaghetti; I replace the meat with flavored tofu or "plant-based ground beef."

If I feel like burgers, hot dogs, or ham sandwiches, I replace the meat with beyond meat beef patties, vegetarian sausages, veggie pates, or vegan "ham."

If I want to make a chicken rice stir-fry, I use the same recipe, but I swap the chicken with vegan chicken pieces.

As for milk, many dairy-free milk variants are now available such as almond or oat milk.

For cheese we now have dairy-free cheese available that tastes just as good as the dairy option.

Fish? Vegan sushi is delicious, and frozen vegan fish fingers are just as tasty as the original ones.

Eggs? You can scramble and flavor tofu to look and tastes like eggs. Some companies have now come out with alternatives with textures, look and taste that are so similar to eggs, you could probably not tell the difference. It has never been easier to go vegan!

Where do you get iron from?

Green leafy vegetables, beans, legumes, seeds, whole grains, nuts and dried fruit contain plenty of iron. On top of it, a vegan diet is plentiful of fruit and vegetables packed with Vitamin C, which helps the body absorb iron.

We are omnivores.

Could you eat raw chicken? Raw pig? Could you eat a carcass? Why not then? Have you ever witnessed any other carnivores or omnivores BBQ in the wild? No, only humans with their big brains have learned to process meat through heat to kill harmful bacteria that would otherwise make them sick. It has been beneficial to our survival adding new sources of food in environments where resources were scares, but it is not making us carnivores or omnivores for it, we are "cheating" plant eaters.

Will I need to supplement calcium if I don't eat dairy?

The dairy industry is selling this calcium myth because they want you to keep drinking cow milk. Calcium is found in green leafy veggies such as broccoli, kale, cabbage, and watercress. Dried fruits, nuts, seeds, and legumes are also excellent sources of calcium. Many vegan milk alternatives also contain adequate levels of calcium.

Where do you get B12 vitamins?

Vegans can find their vitamin B12 in Tempeh (fermented soybeans), nutritional yeast, marmite, B12 fortified plant-based milk, ready to eat cereals, and many other fortified foods. Read the labels as many vegan prepared foods just like non-vegan, are often fortified with the vitamin.

We are top predators like lions; it is natural to eat meat.

When hungry, lions don't open a fridge to eat clean, fresh pieces of meat. They don't need to BBQ their carcasses to digest it either. In other to survive, they must hunt with their own body and eat their catch whole and raw; flesh, organs, fur, guts, skin, bones. That's natural, that's a top predator.

I only buy free-range eggs from happy hens.

Free-range eggs mean having thousands of hens crammed into one big cage instead of thousands of hens crammed in thousands of cages. Same cruelty, different name. Don't fall for it.

If we don't eat farmed animals what will you do with them as they cannot survive in the wild?

Farmed animals are farmed. No demand, no more farming. Yes, it is that simple.

Vegans are extremists.

Imprisoning, raping, killing, torturing or polluting for the selfish pleasure of eating an animal's corpse is very extreme. Eating plants and showing compassion to animals is not.

I only eat fish.

Eating fish is just as destructive, cruel, and unsustainable as meat. If seven billion people turn to fish, our already depleted ocean's fish stock will quickly collapse.

I only eat chicken.

Chicken suffers just as much as any other species. In what way is it more acceptable?

Veganism is a cult, it's like a religion. People shouldn't shove their opinion down my throat.

Are people defending women's rights or child protection shoving their opinion down your throat? Is racial equality a cult? Is social justice a religion? Aren't chains like McDonald's bombarding you with their McNuggets ads?

Vegans have nothing to profit from. Vegans promote their views because they have connected with animals and their suffering. They speak up out of compassion. If you were the victim, you would like people to speak up for you. Vegans are the only voice animals have.

What's wrong with eggs and dairy?

In terms of cruelty, the female animals abused for such food suffer longer than their male counterparts. They all eventually end up in a slaughterhouse, only after extended misery.

Plants have feelings too.

If you are so concerned with plant feelings, stop eating meat. Most crops on earth are fed to farmed animals.

I could never give up cheese!

Yes, you can, it's a decision, and it's easier than most imagine. The cruelty involved in making cheese is not worth it. If producing cheese involved abusing children, would you still eat it? So how much torture are your taste buds worth? We are better than this.

Shouldn't you care about humans first?

Veganism is caring for humans too in providing more food resources for all and protecting humanity's only planet. Caring for animals doesn't stop you from caring for humans.

I know vegans and vegetarians that have no energy and are very pale.

I also know meat-eaters with low energy and pale skin. Poor food habits can either be meat or plant based. If you only eat salads all day, you will face health issues just as much as if you only feed on chicken wings. As a plant-based endurance athlete, I could not compete in a 16 hour-long triathlon if I was nutrient deficient.

I only eat local or organic meat.

Organic, local, or any other feel-good marketing catchphrase doesn't change the facts. It still results in taking animal lives, polluting the Earth, and maintaining food insecurity. The Earth cannot produce enough meat to feed seven billion people and counting. Ninety-eight percent of the meat consumed comes from factory farming.

We need to test on animals to save sick children.

The best way to successfully test new drugs and save more children's lives would be to test on humans. Why aren't we doing it then? The answer is simply because it would be totally immoral to do so. Even to harden criminals or serial killers we could not exercise such cruelty, torment or torture called vivisection. Based on the same morality principle, we have no rights or excuses to shamefully abuse defenseless animals for our own gain. Human illnesses belong to humans, not other species.

Eating vegan is expensive.

Meat and dairy products are far more expensive than plant-based food. Generally speaking, nuts are the most expensive part of a vegan diet.

22. NUTRIENTS

"The most ethical diet just so happens to be the most environmentally sound diet, and just so happens to be the healthiest."

Dr. Michael Greger

Let's start with an overlook of nutrient categories before I suggest you a whole week of different vegan meals. The meal plan, along with the vegan pantry staples start at the next chapter if you feel like jumping right in.

From my experience, learning the basics about nutrients is key to a healthy transition towards veganism. It will help you choose your food in a way to maximize and balance your nutrient intake. You will get the best out of your new plant-based way of life.

Macronutrients

Macronutrients are needed in larger quantities (in gram range). They include water, carbohydrates, fat, and protein. Macronutrients (except water) are also called energy-providing nutrients. Energy is measured in calories and is essential for the body to grow, repair, and develop new tissues, conduct nerve impulses, and regulate life process.

- **Carbohydrates**

  Provide the body's primary source of energy (four calories per gram); they form the major part of stored food in the body for later use of energy and exist in three forms: sugar, starch, and fiber. The brain works entirely on glucose alone. When in excess, it is stored in the liver as Glycogen. Carbohydrates are also essential for fat oxidation and can also be converted into protein.

- **Fats**

  Are used in making steroids and hormones and serve as solvents for hormones and fat-soluble vitamins. Fats have the highest caloric content and provide the most significant amount of energy when burnt. When measured by a calorimeter, fats provide about nine calories per gram of fat, making them twice as energy-rich than protein and carbohydrates. Extra fat is stored in adipose tissue and is burnt when the body has run out of carbohydrates.

- **Proteins**

  They provide amino acids and make up most of the cell structure, including the cell membrane. They are the last to be used of all macronutrients. In cases of extreme starvation, the muscles in the body, that are made up of proteins, are used to provide energy. This is called muscle wasting. As for carbohydrates, proteins also provide 4 calories per gram.

- **Water**

  Makes up a large part of our body weight and is the main component of our body fluids. The body needs more water every day than any other nutrient, and we replenish it through foods and liquids we eat and drink. Water serves as a carrier, distributing nutrients to cells and removing wastes through urine. It is also a compulsory agent in the regulation of body temperature and ionic balance of the blood. Water is essential for the body's metabolism and is also required for lubricant and shock absorber.

Micronutrients

These nutrients include minerals and vitamins. Unlike macronutrients, these are required in very minute amounts. Together, they are extremely important for the normal functioning of the body. Their primary function is to enable the many chemical reactions to occur in the body. Micronutrients do not function for the provision of energy.

- **Vitamins**

  Essential for normal metabolism, growth and development, and regulation of cell function. They work together with enzymes and other substances that are necessary for a healthy life. Vitamins are either fat-soluble or water-soluble. Fat-soluble Vitamins can be stored in the fatty tissues in the body when in excess. Water-soluble vitamins are excreted in urine when in excess and so need to be taken daily.

Water-soluble vitamins include Vitamin B, and C. Green leafy vegetables are rich in Vitamin B, whereas Vitamin C is found abundantly in citrus fruits. Fat-soluble vitamins are Vitamin A, D, E, and K. Green leafy vegetables and plant oils provide these vitamins.

B12 is an essential vitamin linked to the production of red cells, among other functions. It is important for vegan to pay attention to it as we do not find it in plants. Vegans can find their vitamin B12 in Tempe (fermented soybeans), yeast, marmite, and B12 fortified plant-based milk, ready to eat cereals and many other fortified foods. Read the labels as many vegan prepared foods, (just like non-vegan) are often fortified with the vitamin.

- **Minerals**
  are found in an ionized form in the body. They are further classified into macrominerals and microminerals (or trace minerals). Macrominerals present in the body include Calcium, Potassium, Iron, Sodium, and Magnesium, to name a few. Iron is a constituent of Hemoglobin which is present in the blood. Macrominerals are needed in more amounts, as compared to microminerals. Microminerals include Copper, Zinc, Cobalt, Chromium, and Fluoride. They are mostly co-factors and are necessary for the function of enzymes in the body but are needed only in minor quantities. Approximately 4% of the body's mass

consists of minerals.

Daily Intake

To know precisely how much of each nutrient you need every day, I suggest you get professional advice as this may vary with your lifestyle, body weight, age and gender

The estimated amounts of calories needed to maintain energy balance vary with gender, age groups, and different levels of physical activity. But as a rule of thumb, the average person needs about 2000 Calories per day. If you eat more calories than your body needs, you'll gain weight. Eat fewer calories than required, and you will lose weight.

- **Protein**

  You need to get 10 to 35 percent of your calories from protein. This means you'll need roughly 50 to 145 grams of protein each day. Protein requirements are based on body weight. To figure out the minimum amount of protein you need, multiply 0.8 grams of protein by your weight in kilograms. If you don't know your weight in kilograms, find it by dividing your weight in pounds by 2.2. (0.36 grams of protein per pound.)

- **Carbohydrates**

  The average 2000 calorie diet should contain between 210 and 290 grams of carbohydrates each day, which is equal to 45 to 65 per cent of your daily calories. Many people are surprised to learn that the need for carbohydrates is so high it's about half of your daily calories! Since carbohydrates are the main source of energy for the body and brain, they are an important component of a healthy diet. Carbohydrates are not technically essential to your diet since the body can make fuel from fat and protein. However, removing carb-rich foods could result in fiber, vitamin and mineral deficiencies.

Complex Carbohydrate
These come from vegetables, grains (such as bread, pasta, cereal), some fruits, seeds, nuts and legumes (like beans and lentils)

Nutrient-poor simple Carbohydrate
Refined sugars (For an optimal diet, limit your intake of nutrient-poor simple carbohydrates.)

Nutrient-rich simple Carbohydrate
Comes from fruits

Fiber Carbohydrate
Comes from whole grains, vegetables, fruits, seeds, nuts and legumes

- **Fiber**
  Fiber is a non-digestible carbohydrate, which means that our body does not break it down. Instead, the fiber creates intestinal bulk and helps keep our bowels moving regularly. Aim for 30-40 grams of fiber each day.

- **Fat**
  Fat is a nutrient. It is crucial for normal body

function, and without it, we could not live. Not only does fat supply us with energy, it also makes it possible for other nutrients to do their jobs. The average 2000 calorie diet should have between 40 and 65 grams of fat per day (20 to 35 per cent of calories).

Fats, which consist of a wide group of compounds, are usually soluble in organic solvents and insoluble in water. There are different types of fats, which are considered good and bad. Let's see what foods they can be found in.

Oils
Any fat that exists in liquid form at room temperature. Oils are also any substances that do not mix with water and have a greasy feel.

Animal fats
Butter, lard, cream, fat in (and on) meats.

Vegetable fats
Olive oil, peanut oil, flax seed oil or corn oil for instance.

Fats or fatty acids
This refers to all types of fat. However, fats are commonly referred to as those that are solid at room temperature.

Lipids
All types of fats, regardless of whether they are

liquid or solid. Lipids are an essential part of the diet of all humans and many types of animals. Fat is stored in the body for many reasons like vitamin storage; it is not only for energy reserve.

▪ Types of fat

Since fat is a popular topic in diets, let's take a closer look at the different types of fats and what they imply.

Saturated fats

They are solid at room temperature and are sometimes called solid fat. They are saturated, meaning that each molecule of fat is covered in hydrogen atoms.

Saturated fats increase health risks if a person consumes too much over a long period. A large intake of saturated fats may eventually raise cholesterol levels, which increases the risk of cardiovascular disease and stroke.

Where is saturated fat found?

The highest levels of saturated fats can be found in meat (mammals), meat products, the skin of poultry, dairy products, many processed foods, such as cakes, biscuits, pastries, and chips, as well as coconut oil, palm oil, and cocoa butter.

A healthy diet includes less than 10 percent of its calories from saturated fats. Examples of healthy replacement foods would be nuts, seeds, avocado, beans, and vegetables.

Unsaturated fats

Unsaturated fats, which include monounsaturated and polyunsaturated fats, are liquid at room temperature. They are mostly derived from plant oils and classified as "good" fats.

Monounsaturated fats

Monounsaturated fat molecules are not saturated with hydrogen atoms - each fat molecule has only the space for one hydrogen atom.

Monounsaturated fats may lower LDL (low-density lipoprotein - bad) cholesterol and keep HDL (high-density lipoprotein - good) cholesterol at higher levels. But, unless saturated fat intake is reduced, cholesterol levels may remain unchanged.

Many health professionals, however, say that these fats might still reduce a person's risk of developing heart disease. For instance, the Mediterranean diet, a well-researched and chronic disease-risk lowering diet, is full of monounsaturated fats.

You can find monounsaturated fats from many sources like nuts and seeds, avocados, soybean, rice bran, olives or cooking oils made from plants.

Polyunsaturated fats

In polyunsaturated fats, there are a number of spaces around each polyunsaturated fat molecule -

they are not saturated with hydrogen atoms.

Nutritionists say that polyunsaturated fats are good for our health, especially those known as omega-3 polyunsaturated fatty acids.

Omega-3 fatty acids protect against heart disease by lowering blood cholesterol levels and possibly inflammation. Healthcare professionals say omega-3 polyunsaturated fatty acids may also help reduce the symptoms experienced by people who suffer from arthritis, joint problems in general, and some skin diseases.

The other type of polyunsaturated fats is omega-6 fatty acids. These are mostly found in vegetable oils and processed foods. Excessive intake of omega-6's, which is common in the standard American diet, may lead to increased inflammation.

Here are some foods containing Omega 3 polyunsaturated fats in a vegan diet; chia seeds, brussels sprout, algal oil (from seaweeds), hemp seeds, walnuts, flaxseeds, safflower, grapeseed or soybean.

Trans fats
Trans fats are synthetically made, they do not naturally occur. Trans fats are created in an industrial process that adds hydrogen to liquid vegetable oils to make them more solid. They are also known as partially hydrogenated oils.

Trans fats are not essential for human life, and they most certainly do not promote good health. Consuming trans fats increases LDL cholesterol level and lowers levels of HDL cholesterol; this, in turn, raises the risk of developing coronary heart disease and stroke about three times higher than other fats.

The Harvard School of Public Health estimates that trans-fat intake is associated with 50,000 fatal heart attacks each year. They are also associated with an increased risk of developing type 2 diabetes. Experts say that trans fats from partially hydrogenated oils are worse for your health than naturally occurring oils.

Trans fats have become popular because food companies find them easy to use and cheap to produce. They also last a long time and can give food a nice taste. As trans fats can be used many times in commercial fryers, they are commonly used in fast food outlets and restaurants. Several cities and states, including New York City, Philadelphia, and California, have banned or are in the process of banning trans fats.

Where are trans fats commonly found?
Fried foods, such as French fries, doughnuts, pies, pastries, biscuits, pizza dough, cookies, crackers, stick margarines, shortenings, packaged foods, fast foods, and many other baked foods. If nutritional

labeling includes partially hydrogenated oils, it means that food has trans fats.

The American Heart Association says that consumption of trans fats should not exceed 5-6 percent of total calorie intake, though any amount, even if small, increases risk for various health problems.

The take-home message is that not all fats are equal. Staying informed and reading the labels can help you make good dietary choices and replace unhealthy fats with healthy fats and fibrous plants.

*If you would like to know the specific nutrient content of certain foods, you can visit tools.myfooddata.com where you can get each nutritional value separately. *

CONGRATS!

Learning about nutrients and health issues is a little technical, but you are giving yourself the tools to thrive on a vegan diet. Do not hesitate to come back to the nutrient section of the book. I regularly do it myself to refresh my memory. The more comfortable you will be with the data, the better and easier your grocery list will be.

Personal tip on Supplements

If you live a busy life and you don't always have time to cook or if cooking isn't your thing and you resort many time a week on prep meals or restaurants, I suggest you take a portion of "Vega" every other day to boost your nutrient intake. Compare to "centrum" or popular supplements

Vega is made from carefully selected plant-based food ingredients you'd choose yourself if you had the time.

Vega was formulated by Branden Brazier a former Ironman triathlete (1998–2004). Winner of the Canadian 50k division of the Harriers Elk/Beaver National Ultramarathon Championships in 2003 and the 50 km division of the Toronto Ultra Race in 2006.

23. VEGAN PANTRY STAPLES

To help you prepare your one-week meal plan or many other vegan recipes, you'll need basic ingredients you may not have already in your kitchen. These ingredients should be available at most grocery stores.

Buy the organic version of your food, whenever possible. Contrary to conventional practices, organic agriculture is a production system that regenerates the health of soils, ecosystems, and people.

Organic farming relies on natural processes, biodiversity, and cycles, adapted to local conditions rather than the use of synthetic inputs like chemical fertilizers, pesticides, and herbicides. GMOs are not allowed in organic cultures.

Buying organic is always an investment worth doing towards your health and the ecosystem.

Grains

- Quinoa
- Steel-cut oats
- Couscous
- Brown rice

- Barley
- Amaranth
- Whole-Wheat Pasta

Proteins

- Dried or canned beans
- Dried or canned chickpeas
- Dried or canned lentils
- Dried or canned split peas
- Tofu*
- Tempeh*
- Raw cashews
- Walnuts
- Raw almonds
- Pumpkins seeds
- Hemp seeds

Baking

- Whole wheat flour
- Almond meal
- Agave nectar
- Molasses
- Maple syrup
- Organic cane sugar
- Flaxseed
- Chia seeds
- Dairy-free chocolate chips

- Cacao powder
- Medjool dates

Cooking

- Olive oil
- Sesame oil
- Coconut oil
- Liquid aminos
- Balsamic vinegar
- Red wine vinegar
- Apple cider vinegar
- Vegetable broth
- Cornstarch
- Dried mushrooms
- Miso paste
- Tomato paste
- Siracha
- Spices
- Agar-Agar powder

Canned Goods & Miscellaneous

- Diced or crushed tomatoes
- Marinara sauce
- Tamari
- Tahini
- Nut butter
- Unsweetened applesauce

- Coconut milk
- Almond milk
- Canned pumpkin
- Nutritional yeast (B12 enriched)
- Vegan mayonnaise

24. Vegan One-Week Meal Plan

If you ever wondered what vegans eat on a daily basis, you will find here a pretty good sample. This delicious one-week meal plan you can find on PETA's web site, proposes three different dishes and one snack per day.

Made with simple, affordable ingredients, that's 28 different easy to make recipes to kick in your new plant-based way of life. You can go the classic way and use this chapter like a cooking book or have a look online following the web link at the bottom of each recipe.

If you would like to learn more about vegan cooking and recipes, I suggest you visit the vegan chef Jean-Philippe Cyr's page at www.thebuddhistchef.com.

Let's get started!

Day 1   One-Week Meal Plan

Avocado Toast with Garbanzo Beans

(Makes 1 serving)

Ingredients

1 large avocados
1/2 cup cherry tomatoes
1/4 cup garbanzo beans
1/2 lemon
1 Tbsp. olive oil

1 Tbsp. parsley
1 tsp. red pepper flake
Salt and pepper to taste
2 slices whole grain
bread

Instructions

1. Slice avocado in half and remove the pit. Cut into cubes and pour the cubes into a bowl. Add salt and pepper, and squeeze lemon juice into the bowl. Mix thoroughly.

2. Begin to toast the bread. Once the bread is toasted, drizzle olive oil on the bread before adding other ingredients.

3. Scoop the avocado mixture onto the bread.

4. Garnish with cherry tomatoes, garbanzo beans, minced parsley, and red pepper flakes.

www.peta.org/recipes/avocado-toast-garbanzo-beans

Day 1 One-Week Meal Plan
_____

LUNCH

Strawberry-Almond-Kale Salad with Citrus Vinaigrette

(Makes 3 to 4 serving)

Ingredients

1 bunch kale, stemmed
1 lb. strawberries, sliced
1/4 cup sliced almonds
Juice of 1 lemon
2 Tbsp. olive oil
1 Tbsp. agave

1/8 tsp. salt
1/8 tsp. black pepper
3-4 Tbsp. orange juice
(optional)

Instructions

1. Tear the kale into bite-sized pieces and massage with your hands until soft, about 30 seconds. (This makes the kale easier to eat.)

Place in a bowl and add the strawberries and almonds.

2. To make the dressing, combine the lemon juice, olive oil,

agave, salt, and pepper and pour over the salad. For an extra kick, splash orange juice over the salad and enjoy.

www.peta.org/recipes/strawberry-almond-kale-salad-with-citrus-vinaigrette

Day 1   One-Week Meal Plan

DINNER

Tofu-Spinach Lasagna

(Makes 6 to 8 servings)

Ingredients

1/2 lb. lasagna noodles 2 10-oz. packages frozen chopped spinach, thawed and drained
1 lb. soft tofu
1 lb. firm tofu
1 Tbsp. sugar

1/4 cup soymilk
1/2 tsp. garlic powder
2 Tbsp. lemon juice
3 tsp. minced fresh basil
2 tsp. salt
4 cups tomato sauce

Instructions

1. Cook the lasagna noodles according to the package directions. Drain and set aside.

2. Preheat the oven to 350 degrees F.

3. Squeeze the spinach as dry as possible and set aside.

4. Place the tofu, sugar, soymilk, garlic powder, lemon juice, basil, and salt in a food processor or blender and blend until smooth. Stir in the spinach.

5. Cover the bottom of a 9-inch-by-13-inch baking dish with a thin layer of tomato sauce, then a layer of noodles (use about one-third of the noodles). Follow with half of the tofu filling. Continue in the same order, using half of the remaining tomato sauce and noodles and all of the remaining tofu filling. End with the remaining noodles, covered by the remaining tomato sauce. Bake for 25 to 30 minute.

www.peta.org/recipes/tofu-spinach-lasagne/

Day 1   One-Week Meal Plan

SNACK

Fresh veggies and hummus

Day 2

One-Week Meal Plan

Healthy Triple-Layer Smoothie

(Makes 3 serving)

Ingredients

3 cups banana chunks, frozen
1 20-oz. can pineapple chunks, juice reserved

1/2 cup kale or spinach leaves
1/2 cup raspberries
1 cup blueberries

Instructions

1. Add 1 cup of the frozen banana chunks and 1 cup of the pineapple chunks to a blender and blend until smooth. Divide evenly among 3 glasses.

2. Blend together another cup of the frozen banana chunks, 1/2 cup of the pineapple chunks, and the kale or spinach. Add some pineapple juice, if needed, to keep things moving. Carefully add to the glasses, trying not to

mix the colors.

3. Blend together the remaining cup of frozen banana chunks with the raspberries and blueberries. Add some pineapple juice, if needed. Carefully pour into the glasses and serve immediately.

www.peta.org/recipes/recipes/detox-smoothie/

Day 2   One-Week Meal Plan

LUNCH

Vegan Battered 'Fish' Tacos

(Makes 6 tacos)

Ingredients

1 pkg. Gardein fishless filets (https://www.gardein.com/products/golden-fishless-filet/)
1 tsp. oil or lime juice
6 medium-sized corn tortillas
1/2 cup guacamole or 1 avocado, sliced
Diced onion (optional)
chopped cilantro (optional)
jalapeño slices (optional)
lime juice (optional)

Instructions

1. Cook the fishless filets according to package directions.

2. Warm the oil in a pan over medium heat. Place a tortilla in the pan and cook, turning once, until softened.

3. Remove from the pan and spread with 1 tablespoonful of the guacamole.

4. Cut the cooked fishless filets into strips and place 3 strips on the tortilla. If desired, top with diced onion, chopped cilantro, and jalapeño slices and drizzle with

lime juice.

5. Repeat with the remaining tortillas.

6. Serve with salsa, and vegan sour cream.

www.peta.org/recipes/fish-tacos/

Day 2   One-Week Meal Plan

DINNER

Vegan Macro Bowl

(Makes 2 servings)

Ingredients

1/2 lb. extra-firm tofu, drained, pressed, and cubed
1 Tbsp. olive oil
1 Tbsp. soy sauce
Pinch basil
Pinch oregano
1 cup cooked brown rice

1 Tbsp. miso paste
1/2 bunch broccoli, cut into florets and steamed
1/2 cooked sweet potato, diced
1 large carrot, shredded
1 tsp. sauerkraut
1 tsp. pickled ginger (optional)

Instructions

1. Combine the tofu, olive oil, soy sauce, basil, and oregano in a pan and cook on medium heat until the tofu is browned.

2. Mix the cooked brown rice and miso paste together in a medium-sized bowl. Add the tofu mixture, broccoli, sweet potato, carrot, sauerkraut, and pickled ginger and enjoy

www.peta.org/recipes/ vegan-macro-bowl/

Day 2   One-Week Meal Plan

SNACK

Popcorn with nutritional yeast

www.peta.org/living/food/nutritional-yeast-only-sounds-gross

Day 3   One-Week Meal Plan

BREAKFAST

Classic Potato Pancakes

(Makes 6-8 servings)

Ingredients

3 lbs. baking potatoes, peeled

1 yellow onion, finely chopped

Egg Replacer equivalent
of 2 eggs (such as Ener-
G Egg Replacer)
1 tsp. salt

1/4 tsp. pepper
4 Tbsp. unbleached flour
Oil for frying

Instructions

1. Grate the potatoes
and squeeze out the
moisture. In a large
mixing bowl, combine
the potatoes with all the
remaining ingredients,
except the oil.

2. Heat 1/4 cup oil in a
large skillet. Place 3
Tbsp. of the mixture into
the skillet for each latke.

Use a spatula to flatten
the mixture to form the
latke.

3. Fry over medium heat
about 4 minutes per side,
or until golden brown.

4. Drain on paper towels
and serve hot with apple
sauce or soy sour cream.

www.peta.org/living/food/classic-potato-pancakes/

Day 3 One-Week Meal Plan

Black Bean Veggie Burgers

(Makes 6 serving)

Ingredients

1/2 onion (chopped small)
1 (14-ounce) can black beans (well-drained)
2 slices bread (crumbled)
1/2 Tbsp. seasoned salt

1 Tbsp. garlic powder
1 Tbsp. onion powder
1/2 cup flour
Dash salt (or to taste)
Dash pepper (or to taste)
Oil for frying (divided)

Instructions

1. To a small frying pan over medium-high heat, add just enough oil to grease the bottom. Add the onions and sauté them until they are soft - about 3 to 5 minutes.

2. In a large bowl, mash the beans until almost smooth.

3. Add the sautéed onions to the mashed black beans, along with the crumbled bread, seasoned salt, garlic powder, and onion powder, mixing to combine well.

4. Add the flour a few Tbsp. at a time and mix to combine well. Your veggie burger mixture will be very thick (you may want to use your hands to work the flour in well).

5. Form the black bean mixture into individual patties, approximately 1/2-inch thick. The best way to do this is to roll a handful into a ball, then gently flatten it.

6. Fry your black bean patties in a small amount of oil over medium-low heat until slightly firm and lightly browned on each side, about 3 minutes. If your pan is too hot, your bean burgers will brown too quickly and not be heated through and cooked in the middle, so adjust the heat as needed.

7. To serve, assemble your veggie burgers and enjoy with all the fixings. Or, serve them on a plate to with a little ketchup or hot sauce and no bun. A nice green salad can round this out into a nutritious meal.

www.peta.org/recipes/buddhist-chefs-black-bean-veggie-burger

Day 3

One-Week Meal Plan

Enchilada Pie

(Makes 6 to 8 servings)

Ingredients

1/2 tube Soyrizo
2 15-oz. cans beans
(refried or whole)
20 tortillas
1 pkg. vegan cheese
shreds
1 bottle enchilada sauce
Green onions, for

topping (optional)
Black olives, for topping
(optional)
Vegan chipotle aioli
(optional)
Vegan sour cream
(optional)

Instructions

1. Preheat the oven to 400°F.

2. In a large bowl, mix the Soyrizo and beans.

3. In a round baking dish, layer the tortillas, Soyrizo mixture, and vegan cheese. Alternate the three layers until you run out of tortillas, but make sure that your top layer is a tortilla.

4. Pour the enchilada sauce over the stacked pie, top with vegan

cheese, and bake for 20 minutes. Allow to cool for 10 minutes.

5. Garnish with desired toppings, cut into quarters, and enjoy!

www.peta.org/recipes/enchilada-pie/

Day 3   One-Week Meal Plan

SNACK

Spicy Buffalo Cauliflower 'Wings'

(Makes 4 servings)

Ingredients

1 cup water or soy milk
1 cup flour (any kind will work—even gluten-free!)
2 tsp. garlic powder
1 head of cauliflower,

chopped into pieces
1 cup buffalo or hot sauce
1 Tbsp. vegetable oil or melted vegan butter

Instructions

1. Preheat the oven to 450°F.

2. Combine the water or soymilk, flour, and garlic

powder in a bowl and stir until well combined.

3. Coat the cauliflower pieces with the flour

mixture and place in a shallow baking dish. Bake for 18 minutes.

4. While the cauliflower is baking, combine your buffalo sauce and olive oil or margarine in a small bowl.

5. Pour the hot sauce mixture over the baked cauliflower and continue baking for an additional 5 to 8 minutes.

6. Serve alongside vegan blue cheese dressing and celery sticks.

www.peta.org/recipes/spicy-buffalo-cauliflower-wings/

Day 4   One-Week Meal Plan

BREAKFAST

Red bell peppers and hearty kale tofu scramble

(Makes 4 servings)

Ingredients

2 Tbsp. canola oil, or
high heat oil of choice
1 small (8 ounce/227
gram) russet potato,
diced into about 1/2
inch pieces
1 medium onion, diced
1 bell pepper (any color),
cut into strips
3 garlic cloves, minced
1 (14 ounce/400 gram)
package extra firm tofu,
drained and patted dry
2 cups sliced kale leaves
2 Tbsp. soy sauce

2 Tbsp. nutritional yeast
flakes
1 tablespoon ground
cumin
1 Tbsp. turmeric
1 tablespoon hot sauce
(Cholula works well), or
to taste
Black pepper, to taste
Kala namak, to taste
(optional - for eggy
flavor)
Toppings or
accompaniments of
choice

Instructions

1. Coat the bottom of a
large skillet with the oil
and place it over
medium heat.

2. Give the oil a minute
to heat up, and when it
begins to shimmer add
the potatoes and onions.

3. Cook the potatoes and
onions, flipping

occasionally, until the
potatoes are fork tender
and crisp on the outside,
and the onions are soft
and browned, about 10
minutes.

4. Add the bell pepper.
Cook about another two
minutes, until the pepper
begins to soften up.

5. Push everything to the sides of the skillet and add the garlic to the middle. Cook the garlic for about 1 minute, until very fragrant.

6. Break tofu into bite-sized chunks and add it to skillet. Flip everything a few times with a spatula to mix the ingredients.

7. Cook for about 5 minutes, flipping occasionally, until the tofu begins to dry up and crisp in spots.

8. Add the kale, in batches if needed, letting each batch wilt slightly before adding the next.

9. Stir in the soy sauce, nutritional yeast, cumin, and turmeric. Flip everything again to incorporate the ingredients. Cook for 1 to 2 minutes, until most of the soy sauce dries up and the kale has fully wilted.

10. Remove the skillet from heat and season the scramble with hot sauce, kala namak, and black pepper to taste.

11. Serve with toppings and accompaniments of choice.

www.peta.org/recipes/buddhist-chefs-tofu-scramble/

Day 4   One-Week Meal Plan

Vegan Avocado Reuben Sandwich

(Makes 1 sandwich)

Ingredients

2 slices rye or
pumpernickel bread
Mustard Thousand
Island dressing 1/2

avocado, pitted, peeled,
and mashed
1/4 cup sauerkraut

Instructions

1. Spread one slice of bread with some mustard, the other slice with Thousand Island dressing.

2. Place the bread slices, dry side down, in a lightly oiled skillet. Top one slice with avocado, and the other with sauerkraut.

3. Over medium heat, grill the sandwich until lightly browned and hot, about 5 minutes. Put the sandwich halves together and enjoy!

www.peta.org/recipes/avocado-reuben/

Day 4   One-Week Meal Plan

Raw lasagna with walnut meat

(Makes 4 to 6 servings)

Ingredients

1 cup raw cashews, soaked in water for at least 8 hours and drained
1 tsp. salt
2 cloves garlic
1/4 cup nutritional yeast
1 Tbsp. apple cider vinegar or lemon juice
2 medium tomatoes, chopped and seeds removed
2 Tbsp. sundried tomatoes
1 cup raw walnuts
1/2 tsp. fresh rosemary
1/2 tsp. fresh parsley
3–4 zucchini, sliced lengthwise
Basil, for garnish

Instructions

1. In a food processor, blend together the cashews, 1/2 tsp. salt, 1 clove garlic, the nutritional yeast, and the apple cider vinegar or lemon juice. If the mixture is too thick, add water until the desired consistency is reached. Transfer to a bowl and set aside.

2. Add the remaining salt and garlic, fresh tomatoes, sundried tomatoes, walnuts, rosemary, and parsley to the food processor and blend.

3. Lay zucchini slices along the bottom of a greased casserole dish. Spread some of the tomato mixture over top, followed by more zucchini slices, a layer of the cashew mixture, and another layer of zucchini slices. Repeat until you've used up both mixtures and all the zucchini slices.

4. Garnish with basil and serve.

www.peta.org/recipes/delicious-raw-vegan-lasagne/

Day 4   One Week Meal Plan

SNACK

Easy Baked Kale Chips

(Makes 2 servings)

Ingredients

1 qt. chopped kale
1 Tbsp. olive oil

1/4 tsp. salt
1/2 tsp. garlic powder

Instructions

1. Preheat the oven to 300°F.

2. Place the kale in a large mixing bowl and add the olive oil, tossing to coat.

3. Sprinkle with the salt and garlic powder, then toss again.

4. Place in a single layer on a baking sheet and bake for about 15 minutes, or until crispy.

www.peta.org/recipes/kale-chips/

Day 5   One-Week Meal Plan

BREAKFAST

Bagel with peanut butter and bananas

www.peta.org/living/food/7-ways-eat-bagel/

Day 5   One-Week Meal Plan

Tempeh BLT sandwich with vegan bacon

(Makes 2 servings)

Ingredients

1 tsp. olive oil
2 slices of vegan bacon
(try Lightlife Fakin'
Bacon Strips)
2 slices whole grain
bread
1 Tbsp. vegan

mayonnaise
1 small tomato, sliced
Spinach, romaine, or
other dark leafy salad
greens
1/2 avocado, sliced
(optional)

Instructions

1. Heat the olive oil in a
small skillet over
medium heat. Add the
vegan bacon and cook

until golden on both
sides.

2. Meanwhile, toast the

161

bread. Spread with the vegan mayonnaise and top with the "bacon," tomato, greens, and avocado.

www.peta.org/recipes/quick-blt/

Day 5   One-Week Meal Plan

DINNER

Spicy Sesame Noodles

(Makes 4 servings)

Ingredients

2/3 cup (150 g) peanut butter
4 Tbsp. soy sauce
2 cloves garlic, minced
1 green onion, chopped
2 Tbsp. sesame oil
1 tsp. cayenne pepper
1/2 lb. (225 g) linguine, or your favorite pasta
2 Tbsp. toasted sesame seeds
1 cup vegetables of your choice
Fresh cilantro leaves to garnish

Instructions

1. In a saucepan, combine the peanut butter, soy sauce, garlic, and green onion and mix well.

2. Add the sesame oil and cayenne pepper. Heat slowly, whisking until smooth. Add vegetables

3. Meanwhile, cook the linguine according to the package directions. Drain.

4. Place the linguine in a large bowl, add the peanut sauce, and toss to coat. Garnish with the toasted sesame seeds and cilantro.

5. Serve hot or cold.

www.peta.org/recipes/spicy-sesame-noodles/

Day 5   One-Week Meal Plan

SNACK

Three-Ingredient Vegan Ice Cream

Ingredients

1 banana, peeled and
frozen
1 Tbsp. peanut butter

1 tsp. cocoa powder
Additional flavorings
(optional)

Instructions

1. Combine all
ingredients in a food
processor or blender and
mix until well combined
and creamy.

2. If desired, add
additional flavors or
toppings, such as
cookies, fresh fruit,
shredded coconut,
cinnamon, or pieces of
candy.

3. Serve immediately.

www.peta.org/recipes/three-ingredient-vegan-ice-cream/

One-Week Meal Plan

Day 6

BREAKFAST

Egg-free french toast

(Makes 3 servings)

Ingredients

1 cup soy milk
2 Tbsp. flour
1 Tbsp. nutritional yeast flakes
1 tsp. sugar or sweetener of your choice

1 tsp. vanilla
1/2 tsp. salt
Pinch nutmeg
6 slices whole wheat bread

Instructions

1. Mix all the ingredients (except the bread slices) in a shallow bowl.

2. Dip the bread slices into the soy-milk mixture and cook, either on a nonstick griddle until browned on both sides or on a greased cookie sheet in a 400°F oven until golden on both sides, turning once.

www.peta.org/recipes/vegan-french-toast

Day 6

Easiest Vegan Mac 'n' Cheese Ever

(Makes 6 servings)

Ingredients

2/3 cup (150 g) peanut butter

4 Tbsp. soy sauce

2 cloves garlic, minced

1 green onion, chopped

2 Tbsp. sesame oil

1 tsp. cayenne pepper

1/2 lb. (225 g) linguine, or your favorite pasta

2 Tbsp. toasted sesame seeds

1 cup vegetables of your choice

Fresh cilantro leaves to garnish

Instructions

1. Place the garlic, turmeric, salt, nutritional yeast, cashews, and water in a blender. Process until completely smooth.

2. Pour over the pasta and stir. Heat before serving.

www.peta.org/recipes/vegan-macaroni-and-cheese

One-Week Meal Plan

Day 6

DINNER

Eggless cobb salad

(Makes 5 servings)

Ingredients

1 10-oz. bag fresh
spinach
1 cup halved cherry or
grape tomatoes
1 pkg. vegan cheese,
crumbled (we used vegan
bleu cheese)
1 15–oz. can garbanzo
beans, drained and
rinsed
1 6–oz. can black olives,
drained, rinsed, and

sliced
1 medium avocado,
peeled, pitted, and cubed
1 pkg. vegan bacon
1/2 cup vegan
mayonnaise
4 Tbsp. yellow mustard
3 Tbsp. agave
4 servings Tofu Eggs
(www.peta.org/recipes/
tofu-eggs/

Instructions

1. Place the spinach,
tomatoes, vegan cheese,
garbanzo beans, black
olives, avocado, and
Tofu Eggs in a large
bowl.

2. Cook the vegan
chicken strips and vegan
bacon according to
package directions. Once
cooled, crumble and add
to the salad.

3. Combine the vegan mayonnaise, mustard, and agave in a bowl.

Pour over the salad or serve on the side to make a great party dish!

www.peta.org/recipes/vegan-cobb-salad-with-honey-mustard-dressing

Day 6

One-Week Meal Plan

SNACK

Beef' and orzo-stuffed peppers

(Makes 4 servings)

Ingredients

1 cup orzo pasta
4 peppers (green, orange, red, or yellow)
2/3 cup tightly packed fresh parsley
1/4 cup vegan parmesan "cheese"
2 Tbsp. chopped walnuts
1 1/2 tsp. dried basil

1 tsp. salt, divided
1 clove garlic
1/4 cup plus 1 Tbsp. olive oil, divided
12 oz. vegan ground beef-style crumbles
1 medium tomato, seeded and chopped
1 12-oz. jar tomato sauce

Instructions

1. Preheat the oven to 350°F.

2. Cook the orzo pasta according to the directions on the package. Drain and set aside.

3. Fill a large pot with water and bring to a boil. Cut the tops off the peppers (save them) and scrape out the insides, removing the seeds. Place the peppers into the boiling water, simmer for 3 minutes, remove from the water, and invert them onto a paper towel to drain.

4. Place the parsley, soy parmesan, walnuts, basil, 1/2 tsp. of the salt, and the garlic into a food processor and pulse until blended. With the food processor running, slowly add 1/4 cup of the olive oil and continue processing to form a smooth pesto.

5. In a large skillet, brown the beef-style crumbles in the remaining oil over medium heat. Stir in the orzo, pesto, the remaining 1/2 tsp. of salt, and the chopped tomato. Continue cooking, stirring frequently, until the mixture is heated through.

6. Pour the tomato sauce into an 8-inch glass baking dish. Fill the peppers with the "beef" mixture and place them into the baking dish. Put the pepper tops back on and bake for 20 minute

www.peta.org/recipes/beef-orzo-stuffed-peppers

Day 7

One-Week Meal Plan

BREAKFAST

Vegan yogurt with fresh fruit, nuts, and seeds

(Makes 3 servings)

www.peta.org/living/food/get-cultured-with-these-vegan-yogurt-brands

Day 7

One-Week Meal Plan

LUNCH

Raw spicy kale soup with Pumpkin seeds (Pepitas)

(Makes 1 serving)

Ingredients

1/2 cups raw pepitas
3 cups chopped kale, fairly tightly packed
1 1/2 cups water
3 Tbsp. freshly squeezed lemon juice
1/4 cup apple juice
1/2 cup mashed avocado
1 tablespoon peeled and minced ginger
1 Tbsp. seeded and diced hot pepper
1 1/2 Tbsp.s sea salt, or to taste
1/8 Tbsp. ground black pepper
Pinch cayenne pepper
1/4 Tbsp. chipotle chile powder, or 1/2 Tbsp. chile powder, optional
1 tablespoon coconut oil or olive oil, optional
1 tablespoon minced cilantro
1/4 cup minced red bell pepper

Instructions

1. Place the pepitas in a small bowl with ample water to cover. Allow to sit for 15 minutes. Drain and rinse well.

2. Place in a strong blender with all of the remaining ingredients except the cilantro, and red bell pepper, and blend until very creamy.

3. Transfer to a bowl, add the cilantro and stir well. Top with red bell pepper before serving.

www.peta.org/living/food/spicy-kale-soup-pepitas

Day 7

One-Week Meal Plan

General Tso's Tofu

(Makes 4 servings)

Ingredients

For the tofu:

1½ Tbsp maple syrup

2 Tbsp Louisiana hot sauce (such as Crystal)

1 pound regular or firm tofu (450g; drained, pat dry, and cut into 1-inch squares)

1 ½ Tbsp. sesame seeds

2 to 3 Tbsp. cornstarch (depending on how wet the tofu is)

⅓ cup peanut or canola oil (for shallow frying)

For the rest of the dish:

½ Tbsp. ginger (minced)

2 cloves garlic (minced)

7 whole dried Chinese red chili peppers (optional)

½ red bell pepper (cut into large pieces)

½ tablespoon Shaoxing wine

1 cup water or vegetable stock

2 cups broccoli florets

1½ Tbsp. light soy sauce

1 Tbsp. dark soy sauce

2 Tbsp.s rice vinegar

¼ Tbsp. salt

1 tablespoon sugar

½ Tbsp. sesame oil

1½ Tbsp. cornstarch (mixed with 1 tablespoon water)

Instructions

1. Mix the Maple syrup and Louisiana hot sauce in a bowl until well combined. Add the tofu to the bowl, and toss together gently with a spatula until the tofu is well-coated.

2. Next, sprinkle the sesame seeds over the tofu, and toss until evenly distributed. Next, sprinkle the cornstarch over the tofu until lightly coated. If the tofu is still too wet, add a little more cornstarch.

3. Heat 1/3 cup oil in a medium-sized frying pan (we like to use a cast iron skillet) until the oil is about 350F, or when a bamboo chopstick bubbles when inserted into the oil. If you want to make the tofu frying easier, use more oil to achieve a deep fry.

4. Carefully place the tofu pieces into the pan, ensuring that the pieces are not touching, and let fry for about 2 minutes. Turn them over to continue frying on the other side. Work quickly and turn the heat down if you need more time for turning, or if you see they are starting to burn. Continue to cook the tofu until a nice crust is formed, and they turn golden brown (about 4-5 minutes time in total). Transfer the tofu pieces to a sheet pan with a slotted spoon.

5. Heat your wok over medium heat and add 1 tablespoon of the oil left from tofu-frying, and add the ginger. After 10 seconds, add the garlic

and the whole dried chili peppers, and stir for 15 seconds. Next, stir in the red bell peppers and Shaoxing wine.

6. Now add the water or vegetable stock, and let the mixture come up to a boil. Add the broccoli florets.

7. Immediately add the soy sauces, rice vinegar, salt, sugar, and sesame oil. Let the mixture come up to a boil. Immediately add the cornstarch mixture slowly while stirring.

8. The sauce should be thick enough to coat a spoon. Feel free to add more or less of the cornstarch mixture depending on how thick you like your sauce but give it 30 seconds to 1 minute between additions, as it does take some time for the sauce to thicken.

9. Toss in your fried tofu and give everything a quick stir to make sure the tofu is coated. Serve with steamed rice!

www.peta.org/recipes/recipes/buddhist-chefs-general-tsos-tofu/

Day 7   One-Week Meal Plan
_____

Faux-Turkey and 'Cheese' Roll-Up

(Makes about 12 roll-ups)

Ingredients

2 Tbsp. vegan
mayonnaise
2 Tbsp. mustard
1 large piece lavash or 3
large tortillas
1 pkg. Peppered Tofurky
Deli Slices or other

Tofurky Deli Slices of
your choice
1 pkg. Follow Your
Heart American Style
Slices
1 bunch spinach

Instructions

1. Spread the vegan
mayonnaise and mustard
onto the lavash.

2. Add the deli slices,

"cheese," and spinach.

3. Roll tightly lengthwise,
cut into 2-inch pieces,
and serve.

www.peta.org/recipes/recipes/faux-turkey-and-cheese-roll-up

Visit

www.aveganplanet.com

Follow us @aveganplanetposts

Facebook Page AVeganPlanet

Made in the USA
Columbia, SC
23 October 2023

24842014R00107